Praise for *Self Source-ery*

'Lisa is a true visionary for us all, and to read her books has been a transformative experience for me. Her words pierce the heart and the soul. She brings the magic of being human into an awareness that can shift your life in an instant, encouraging you to tap into your personal power creatively, decadently, and with ease. Lisa Lister is a true guide (especially during this most transformative time).'

CARRIE-ANNE MOSS, ACTRESS – *THE MATRIX* SERIES, WIFE, MOTHER, FOUNDER OF ANNAPURNA LIVING

'Lisa is the ultimate nurturer, gently guiding us all back to remembrance. She is a fierce, unwavering force of nature, of feminine power, of love.'

LEANN RIMES CIBRIAN, SINGER-SONGWRITER, GRAMMY AWARD WINNER, AND FOUNDER OF SOUL OF EVERLE

'The discovery of Lisa's work (her book *Witch* fell into my lap in a bookstore in the wrong section – a story for another time) came at a time when I was desperate for an explanation as to how, in my 30s, I had become my own cautionary tale. Once fearless and wild, I had wandered into desolate territory, trying desperately to grow a life in dry ground. Trying desperately to behave. To please. To quieten myself for the benefit of others.

Lisa's medicine saved me. In a very real way. Her work didn't give me answers. It gave me a map, hard truths delivered with love and humour, and the provisions I would need to take the journey to find the place long since forgotten. It gave me her compass until I could find my own.'

LEANNE BEST, ACTRESS – *LINE OF DUTY*, *COLD FEET*, *YOUNG WALLANDER*

'Reading the poetic words of *Self Source-ery* made me feel like my soul was calling itself back home. The words flow like velvet and this book is like a deep, much-needed mental massage. If this is what a witch in the 21st century sounds like, then give me the hat and sign me up. I felt deeply nourished and nurtured by Lisa's words, and thank her for this beautiful creation.'

MAUDE HIRST, ACTOR – *THE VIKINGS*, WRITER, MEDITATOR, FOUNDER OF ENERGYRISE

'For anyone who's ever lived in fear of the chaos of their own body and yet nurtured a deeper desire to surrender to and explore its unending wildness, Lisa Lister's work is like the key that unlocks an ancient door that leads you into a fantasy world that you'd always dreamed about, but had almost given up believing in.

Her writing – like her – is bold, bright, beautiful and lovingly provokes the reader to embrace the fullness of their being; of wanting and asking for more and never apologizing for being too much. Reading her books feels like softening into Mama Earth's loving embrace, being held, and then being reminded that I am her and she is me.'

EVANNA LYNCH, ACTRESS – *HARRY POTTER*, BEST-SELLING AUTHOR OF *THE OPPOSITE OF BUTTERFLY HUNTING*, AND COFOUNDER OF KINDERBEAUTY

'In a world of bossy 'self-help' and Instagram 'spirituality,' Lisa is the real deal. She brings something different, much-needed, and nothing short of life-changing. She is wise and wonderful; her work is genuinely authentic and from the heart. She's mystical in the best possible way, but rooted in the real world – she understands everyday life and the time and money limitations we might have. Not to mention her serious wisdom, delivered in a chatty and fun writing style that reminds me of my favourite magazines growing up, which speaks to me on a personal level that I heart very deeply.

Self Source-ery is not just words on a page: it's a call to action. It's the radical magic we all need. It's an invitation to remember our own magic and reclaim our wild selves, as well as the practical tools to do so. Lisa's guidance in this is empathetic, inclusive, and realistic. It feels like what we all need in this moment. We are so lucky to have Lisa and her work in these wild times.'

ELEANOR WOOD, BEST-SELLING AUTHOR OF *STAUNCH*

SELF
SOURCE-ERY

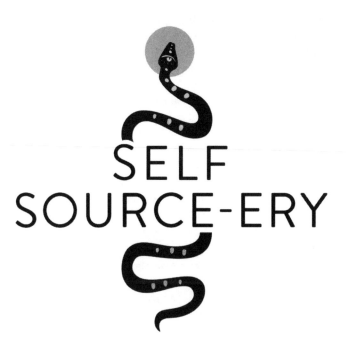

SELF SOURCE-ERY

COME TO YOUR **SENSES**

TRUST YOUR **INSTINCTS**

REMEMBER YOUR **MAGIC**

LISA LISTER

BESTSELLING AUTHOR OF *WITCH*

HAY HOUSE

Carlsbad, California • New York City
London • Sydney • New Delhi

Published in the United Kingdom by:
Hay House UK Ltd, The Sixth Floor, Watson House,
54 Baker Street, London W1U 7BU
Tel: +44 (0)20 3927 7290; Fax: +44 (0)20 3927 7291
www.hayhouse.co.uk

Published in the United States of America by:
Hay House Inc., PO Box 5100, Carlsbad, CA 92018-5100
Tel: (1) 760 431 7695 or (800) 654 5126
Fax: (1) 760 431 6948 or (800) 650 5115
www.hayhouse.com

Published in Australia by:
Hay House Australia Ltd, 18/36 Ralph St, Alexandria NSW 2015
Tel: (61) 2 9669 4299; Fax: (61) 2 9669 4144
www.hayhouse.com.au

Published in India by:
Hay House Publishers India, Muskaan Complex, Plot No.3, B-2,
Vasant Kunj, New Delhi 110 070
Tel: (91) 11 4176 1620; Fax: (91) 11 4176 1630
www.hayhouse.co.in

The information given in this book should not be treated as a substitute
for professional medical advice; always consult a medical practitioner. Any
use of information in this book is at the reader's discretion and risk. Neither
the author nor the publisher can be held responsible for any loss, claim or
damage arising out of the use, or misuse, of the suggestions made, the
failure to take medical advice or for any material on third-party websites.

A catalogue record for this book is available from the British Library.

Tradepaper ISBN: 978-1-78817-757-3
E-book ISBN: 978-1-78817-759-7
Audiobook ISBN: 978-1-78817-758-0

Printed and bound in Great Britain by
TJ Books Limited, Padstow, Cornwall

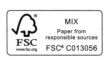

Contents

Setting the Scene

As you read and experience what I share in these pages, you *may* start to smell the fragrance of creation in the air – rose otto, immortelle, bergamot, cinnamon, and ylang-ylang: the essential oil blend that I lovingly applied to my wrists before every writing session.

You *may* be called to find out where Venus and Lilith are in your natal chart (*Self Source-ery* was written during my own 18-month Venus cycle, and well, I'm a Lilith in Leo so the book is infused with BLE – Big Lilith Energy).

You *may* crave rose-infused milk chocolate (I won't lie, *many* bars of this were devoured and savored during the weaving of these words, and there's a good chance I've left behind some chocolate smudges. Sorry about that).

You *may* experience a need, want, desire to scoop pomegranate seeds from a bowl with your fingers and smear and stain your lips a deep and delicious shade of 'pomegranate juice red.' (Yes, pomegranates are rich in symbolism, and they taste good too.)

You *may* want to (and I highly recommend that you do) brew a cup of dream-inducing mugwort tea in your favorite giant mug. (Yep, this book is imbued with the medicine and magic of the mugwort plant. Ma medicine for These Times.) Which is why, as you read, you may – actually, I can pretty much guarantee that you will – also experience what I lovingly call 'the space in-between.' It's dreamy, it's liminal, it's unknown.

Y'see, when I write, I riff. Direct from source, direct from my pelvic bowl – my own bubbling cauldron of creation – with inky red pen into pink Moleskine notebooks. The writing of the book then becomes very much about letting the medicine and magic of those riffs m o o o v e through me, and without too much force, I look to find the patterns. To make meaning – we humans LOVE to make meaning – and for it to become digestible and in some way *useful* to those who read it.

But often, this process can trap what so many of us, especially women, are bloody brilliant at, which is to riff, talk, and create in a spiraling, without beginning or end or a 'known' structure and form, liminal, labyrinth walk kind of way. To let the words and the riffs and the feels and the thrills live and breathe and be experienced through us – spilling, sometimes gushing, messily onto the page, and rarely, if ever, making sense to the thinking mind. (That's because, I believe, Ma wisdom isn't *meant* to be intellectualized.)

So, in this book, I won't try to 'capture' those inky red pen-scribbled notes and confine them to a particular 'structure' as I turn them into shape and form. Instead, like my nanna and mumma before me, I'm going to 'weave.' (They were both the most incredible knitters and weavers of wool. Me? Sadly not, but I'm trying to replicate their skills by collecting the threads to create the whole in word form.)

To weave my own personal mythos with those of the women – real and archetypal – who have gone before and are yet to come. The ever-crossing stories of goddesses, herbs, animal magic, synchronicities, descents and ascents; the dark *and* the light; the oceanic tidal waves of emotion and sensation; the cycles within cycles and my endless fascination with the time-between-times – the cross-quarter days of the Celtic Wheel of the Year, the days of my menstrual cycle when I move from one phase to the next; that time-between-time when we *all* must learn to be in the not knowing.

I want to allow it ALL the space to live and breathe and continue to unfold LONG after you've read it. So that each and every time you return to these pages, you receive something different, deeper. So, my request/invitation/heart call to you is this: Recognize and surrender any/all mechanical/patriarchal conditioning and programming you may have around reading a book simply to receive information, and for that book to be structured in a way that makes 'complete sense' – a 'finished product' that will 'tell' you what to do.

Instead, can you let yourself simply soften to the idea of being open?

Open to receive.

Open to receive *exactly* what you need.

Everything you need to come to your senses, trust your instincts, and remember.

To remember your magic.

To remember you *are* magic.

To experience, hear, smell, see, sense, and witness how the words and magic woven, whispered, sung, and drummed through these pages make *you* f e e e l.

What magic and medicine wants to be remembered THROUGH you?

These Times are wild.
Thankfully, so are you.

What Is Self Source-ery?

It's in the chaos of These Times that I've been called to create and share this book, because chaos *is* the mother of creation. But what exactly is Self Source-ery?

It's super simple, YET thoroughly complex. Yep, as is the way of the feminine – and this book is placed firmly in the realm of feminine magic (because we need it more than ever) – Self Source-ery is paradoxical because there's NOTHING to learn and EVERYTHING to remember. It's archetypal, mythical, and ancient. AND it's real-time, parallel, present, and future. All at the same time.

It's self-love

Only, to avoid the eye rolls that the term 'self-love' often evokes, let's call it you in deep and delicious relationship with your body.

You, with the deepest compassion for yourself, your body, and your experience, returning to and coming into alignment with your true and real nature.

You, recognizing and acknowledging what your needs, wants, and desires are from THAT place.

You, taking fierce responsibility for sourcing those needs, wants, and desires, through your body's wisdom and intelligence, without shame, guilt, or embarrassment.

It's liberation

Self Source-ery unhooks you from the incessant need to seek and strive – the 'what next?' and fear-freakery and the conditioned belief that you need to be 'good' – and it allows you to create a stretchy and permeable container in which *you* get to set boundaries, choose what you believe and align with, fill yourself up, nourish yourself, cultivate your energetics, and remember your magic. The magnetic magic and wisdom that's held cell-deep – to show up, through you and for you.

It's magic – *YOUR* magic

Self Source-ery is awakening to and working with your innate feminine magic, the power of your presence, your creative force, and the cyclical and rhythmic intelligence of your body, the Earth, and the cosmos to create, regenerate, trust, grow, and heal.

It's not a formula, it's a frequency. YOUR unique-to-you frequency.

NOTE: I'm NOT here to teach you any of this. My intention is *always* to simply share and to be a guide-ess supporting YOUR remembrance.

Surrender to it All

Since writing *Witch* (the book where I first shared the Source-ress as an archetypal, energetic force), and, as is the way when you're someone who lives in the mythos and the mystery of *all* things, I've had my own initiation with Her, source.

And one thing I KNOW to be true is that if you declare to source, in a book called *Witch*, 'let's come undone,' you can guarantee that SHE will, by *any* means necessary, ensure that you do indeed, with allllll the fiercest love, *come undone*. That you *will* find yourself in the dark, the chaotic, and the unknown, meeting parts of yourself that... well, you really don't like. (Or have previously tried *really* hard to ignore.)

Old stories and conditioning that have been buried deep in our psyche – all the mistruths about our bodies, our menstrual blood, and who we are. The spell of the 'good girl.' And the fears – ohmyGoddess, the fears. The fear of the repercussions of being someone who draws too much attention to themselves or takes up too much space; the fear of being abandoned for daring to shine too brightly; the fear of being 'punished' for experiencing pleasure, desire, and sensuality.

Yep, when you say, as I did, that 'as witches, we self-source, create ritual and celebrate our bodies so that when others spend time in our presence and wholeness, they remember themselves too,' you can be damn sure that SHE will support you/kick your ass/initiate the shit out of you so that you do *exactly* that.

But first, you have to surrender. You surrender to it all – the pain, the trauma, the stories about who you are that are not and never will be true. And, like the serpent in every tale about notorious and powerful women (well, certainly in those that I choose to read and to tell), you shed. Audaciously. And you keep shedding. Till you're bone deep.

Down to the bones

Ever heard the phrase 'I know it in my bones'? My nanna used to say it, and no one disagreed with her because she DID know it – and by *it*, I mean everything – in her bones. My nanna, who you may have met through my stories about her in other books, was my very own version of La Loba (a mythical woman of the Indigenous American

Pueblo peoples) – the 'witch' who lived on the edge of society and collected the bones of the dead.

La Loba would sing to the bones, and as she sang, they'd begin to fuse. Flesh and fur would appear, and eventually, a wolf would form and run out into the wild. But the bones my nanna collected were animal bones to make broth – a broth that seemed to be boiling on the hob for my entire childhood. (Probably because it was.) She'd sing Irish folk songs over that broth as she stirred it, to ensure that what we ate was infused with good intentions. (Something I continue to do today when I'm making food for myself and others.)

The good news? When we surrender to all that we think we know – when we shed, layer by layer, down to the bone, down into the marrow where blood is made – we're in the deepest, most resonant part of our self. It's here that we can locate and orientate (even in the dark – *especially* in the dark), and we too can, with intention, sing (and dance and drum) back our wildness. Our wild, primal, instinctual, underneath-it-all, real and true mother-loving nature. Our source-ery.

We land in the power of the Earth; we land in our bodies, we land in Mumma Earth. Our bones resonate, together, and we're grounded, rooted into this time and this space. The here and now. Present to our presence.

And when we're bone deep and connected to the dark, rich, fertile soil of the Earth? *Then* we have capacity. S t r e e e e t c h y capacity to stay connected to the magnetic primal force of Mumma Earth through our body, *and* to let our body – more specifically, our pelvic bowl, our center – become a vessel, a sacred container to open to the vastness of *all* that is, simultaneously, at the same time.

Yep, you're able to remember that you're…

A gloriously cyclical, rhythmical, primal, instinctual, magnetic, self-sensory being who's connected to the Earth, *as* Earth, *through* your body.

Connected to divinity *as* divinity *through* your body.

Connected to the cosmos *as* the cosmos, *through* your body.

You remember Ma. The Great Ma. You remember that you have access to billions of years of Ma healing and wisdom IN your body.

S l o o o w l y and with fierce love, you sing back your wild, you reveal what's real, and you remember your magic.

You create capacity

Your capacity to alchemize and metabolize, to recalibrate and regenerate.

Your capacity to acknowledge, trust, and self-regulate your nervous system. And to feel really good about being IN.YOUR.BODY.

Your capacity to locate and sense your deeper, truer needs. To *sense* it all. To sniff it out, track it, map it, taste it, feel, hear, witness, and experience All. Of. The. Things. (Said *and* not said. Seen *and* not seen.)

Your capacity to take fierce self-responsibility, to discern, and to act accordingly.

Your capacity to choose. (*And* to change your mind.)

Your capacity to experience pleasure and joy.

Your capacity to source your own power, authority, and life force.

BE the Source-ress

Look, I won't lie, the Self Source-ery 'process' *can* be gnarly. AND it can also be *really* bloody brilliant. That's what happens when we live in the fullness of our possibility. It's the most potent medicine of all: the ever-unfolding paradoxes that untether us from our often grippy need to control ALL. OF. THE. THINGS. Our need to be 'sure' and to be 'right.'

So that we're able, with the fiercest compassion, to reclaim Lilith. To reclaim Mary Magdalene. To reclaim ALL of the women throughout time and space who were exiled, burned, drowned, maligned, shamed, called mad and hysterical, and punished for who they were and what they knew.

So that we're able, with potency, power, and reverence, to return.

Return it ALL home. To them, to us, to our bodies. To the Earth.

So that we're able to fully embody and become the archetypical, mythical, AND very real Source-ress:

SHE who is charmed AND dangerous and is NOT afraid of the dark.

SHE who trusts herself, her inner sight, her bone-deep wisdom.

SHE who tends to, nourishes, holds, and regulates herself.

SHE who honors and satiates her hunger, needs, wants, and desires without blame, shame, or judgment.

SHE who makes magic and medicine. Possibly the potion kind, but *definitely* the elemental and alchemical metabolizing of ALL things *through* the body kind.

SHE who is able to hold space for multiple possibilities, experiences, and outcomes as we navigate, liberate, create, and thrive on this planet. ALL AT THE SAME TIME.

If *Witch* was the call, then *Self Source-ery* is the response.

It's cell-deep nourishment and regeneration for those who are on this Source-ress path.

It's the ability to metabolize, alchemize, and grieve for the death of What's Been Before and to be a fully-aligned-with-the-Divine cocreator of What Comes Next.

It's an attunement and full and deep integration.

It's magic *and* it's real. (Because magic IS real.)

It's feminine artistry. It's a dance with the Divine.

It's a bit science-y (if you want it to be), and it's a fully lived and felt experience.

It's a recognition of the trauma and/or programmed pain of These Times.

And an ever-fiercer recognition that when we live fully inside our skin as a whole being, we have the power, wisdom, and agency in our bodies – through our return to Ma, our primordial power; our reconnection to her cyclical maps of intelligence; our return to nature and our own real and true nature (as cunning folk/alchemists/magic-makers/witches/wise ones) – to embrace simultaneously the pleasure and pain of this life-living experience and make much-needed source-ery (magic and medicine) for ourselves, each other, and the collective.

Self Source-ery is you, fully sourced, by source, nourished, fully satiated, orientated toward life (while knowing death intimately), following your oracular wisdom – your inner sight and gnostic knowing – and trusting the ever-unfolding revealment of being in your body and living *your* rhythm.

About This Book

This book is a cauldron.

A potent container that sits in the space between my experience and yours. As I write and you read, we'll make medicine. Together.

Let what I share be invitations, possibilities, and opportunities for you to f e e e l, remember, and experience what Self Source-ery is for YOU. (Know that, between every line are whispered incantations of love and magic for you. To receive them, simply place a hand on your heart as you read.)

You may recognize yourself in the stories I share and in the feelings I express. (Or you might not.) A certain phrase, or a reference to a particular goddess or concept may pique your interest. (Or it might not.) And that's my role as guide-ess – not to tell you *what* to do and *how* to do it, but to meet you EXACTLY where you are, and to create a supportive space (because space is grace) for YOU to remember YOUR magic.

One of the perks of being the Creatrix of this particular word-weave is that I get to share through the lens of my own lived experience. I'm a woman perpetually birthing more of her 'real.' A woman living cyclically, a woman claiming Self Source-ery as remembered magic that can be trusted, in *my* body.

When I refer to Divine source, I'll often call her SHE. I talk about wombs and periods and orgasms A LOT. Mainly because I have them (although at one point, a doctor in a white coat *did* threaten to 'whip out' my womb – actual phrase he used) and so I really want to honor and celebrate them.

Now, however *you* identify on the glorious spectrum of being human – whether you have a womb or not, whether you menstruate or not – *everything* I share is offered, with love, to EVERYONE who's interested in deepening their relationship with an embodied, cyclical, living experience.

Our experiences WILL be different, but when we remember our magic *together*, and share our experiences and stories *with* each other, they become a web-weaving of ancient-future frequencies, a new mythos for us ALL to believe in as we actualize new paradigms of care for ourselves, each other, and the collective.

Diving in

As with every book I write, *Self Source-ery* is designed to be read as a stand-alone work. However, it's also a deepening companion to all my other books, which are the foundational spiderweb weaving for the magic and medicine shared in *Self Source-ery*.

You can read *Self Source-ery* in one sitting, slowly, while sipping your favorite libation, or you can use it as an oracle – ask a question and flip open a page to receive wisdom. Your call. I also invite you to keep returning to the book once you've read it, because, like the very best kind of burlesque dancer – think Immodesty Blaize and Perle Noire (my two personal favorites) – she's a tease, and with every read, more will *always* be revealed to you. *Wink.*

The book is organized into three medicine bundles (because three *is* the magic number):

Part I: Come to Your Senses – untangling yourself from the societal spell to reclaim your body, specifically your pelvic bowl, as sacred terrain.

Part II: Trust Your Instincts – self-attunement and trust-building in your innate body wisdom to cultivate connected and magnetic source power.

Part III: Remember Your Magic – cyclical and rhythmic maps and medicine to support you, as Source-ress. So that you're no longer simply surviving but actively thriving. (And flourishing in the most nourished way, at source, by source.)

Within each medicine bundle, you'll find the following features:

IN.YOUR.BODY.MENT® practices

I'm a ceremonialist, so I LOVE ritual, but know that EVERY one of the rituals, in fact *all* the practices, that I share in this book are simply an *invitation*.

They form part of a process called IN.YOUR.BODY.MENT® – a unique and nourishing mix of movement, dance, breath work, and sound practices created and curated by me to support and source your magic through the rhythmic intelligence of your body in connection with nature and the cosmos.

Think of these practices as ways to connect, marker points, opportunities in space and time to feel and sense your source-ery IN.YOUR.BODY, to anchor in what you've experienced, and to honor, revere, and hold sacred the process that you're in.

You can modify them, adding your own juice, words, and magic. (If I ever share anything that I think shouldn't be modified – perhaps a movement or a breath that might cause injury if done incorrectly, or something passed down through my lineage that's super sacred and not to be messed with – I'll let you know, OK? Otherwise, change it up, buttercup.)

Journal prompts

The journal prompts in this book aren't *simply* questions. If you let them, they can also act as psyche prods, an opportunity to get out of your own way, stop 'thinking' and instead, drop in and drop down, IN to your body, and allow your heart and pelvic bowl to explore, wander, and get curious about who you are. Because…

Self-discovery = self-knowing
Self-knowing = self-power

SHE Riffs

SHE Riffs are oracular and devotional wordplay direct from SHE, conjured in the belly of the pythoness and shared *through* me. They have been placed, with love, throughout these pages to support your softening. Let them help you to drop deeper into the cauldron of your own wisdom and knowing.

Source-ery support

My nanna taught me from a young age about the power of herbs and plants to soothe and support. The myrrhophores (in ancient times, these were the temple priestesses who worked specifically with sacred oils and perfumes) and Hildegard von Bingen (a medieval mystic and visionary who worked intimately with the magic and medicine of plants) are the inspiration and mentors in my own herbal medicine practice, and between us, we conjure anointing oils, tinctures, teas, and herbal blends. I share some of these in the book to support your Self Source-ery.

NOTE: When working with herbs and essential oils, I urge you to take fierce self-responsibility. Anything and everything I share is NOT to be used as a substitute for medical advice or to diagnose and treat disease or serious health conditions. If you're pregnant and/or experience allergies, please check and double check which herbs you can and cannot work with.

YOU, self-sourced

These bite-sized, love-infused summaries are reminders of how the medicine and magic I've shared support *you* as Source-ress.

Opening Ceremony – Soften to Receive

Yes, that beat you can hear is the sound of me banging my drum – the one I use in *every* circle, in person and online – inviting you to gather here, in this space and time, and to soften to the possibility of letting what I share with you in these pages be a transmission of love that lets the wild, the magical, and what's real reveal itself to, in, and through you.

Pause.

Be here for a moment.

Place a hand on your heart and connect with your breath – feel it rise and fall – and then soften.

Let yourself be soft.

Let yourself soften and be open to receive.

Feel Mumma Earth beneath you.

SHE's got you. SHE can hold you. SHE can/has/does hold it all.

SHE's Ma. Mumma. SHE.

Creatrix.

A primal force.

Divine source.

SHE is you and you are her.

Pause.

Be here. With her.

Let the reverberation of the sound 'Ma' vibrate through your being as I invite you to be open to receive. To consider this book a love letter, a deep bow, an activation, an incantation, a fire ceremony of love and devotion direct from the space in-between.

A space and place that's between times.

The space between What's Been Before and What Comes Next.

A place where there's NO thing, so EVERY thing is possible.

Creation. Potential. Wisdom. Initiation.

Because it's here, in the space in-between, where the most fully lived and fully felt, wild and sensorial experience of being a human, a woman, a Source-ress – with heavy emphasis on the word *source* – is forged.

SHE who has come to, and is led by, her senses. Curious, ever enquiring, and present to the tantalizing vitality of feeling, experiencing, metabolizing, and alchemizing everything IN and THROUGH her body.

SHE who has recognized that she's become desensitized, disassociated, and distracted because of trauma and fear – societal, familial... All. Of. It. SHE *knows* that this was an act of survival, and slowly, with love, she releases herself from the shackles of blame, shame, and guilt. Unravels her own mysteries, trusts her instincts, and becomes a living mythos.

SHE who is divinely connected to source, as source, and remembers, deep down in her belly and bones, the magic of her body, the Earth, and the cosmos.

This dreaming into being – an exploration, art form, mistress-ry, devotional act – is something I lovingly call Self Source-ery: much-needed magic and medicine for These Times. And to enter into, to immerse yourself in, this feminine artistry is to care less about the facts and w a a a a y more about the feels. Because feeling is healing, and healing is revealing. It's the art of well-being.

It's to let your sense-led curiosity reveal both inner and outer maps – specific to you, direct from source – that provide clues and cues to help you remember that you're alive and deserve not only to exist but to thrive. To bloom and flourish because you KNOW what it is to be supported, nurtured, and nourished. At source. By source. Because you ARE source.

Of course, you may not know and remember any of this with your conscious mind. Your made-from-the-starry-stuff self comes into human form and it's so easy to forget – to let the societal spell distract you from reconnecting, rooting, and recalibrating with your inner compass, your own true north: source.

But that's the whole point of *Self Source-ery*, and of every book I write: to get underneath the surface of all that we've been told and sold about who we're supposed to be. To support you in remembering who you *actually* are and what it is you already *know*, deep down in the belly of the pythoness: your sensual, instinctual wildness.

Your source-ery.

Your You-ness. Your potent and powerful medicine and magic.

It's what the world so desperately needs the most right now.

But you already know that, right? That's why you're here.

I'm sure that you'd be the first to admit that you've already eaten, occasionally overindulged, at the spiritual buffet of wellness and new age – I mean, haven't we all? And yet there's *still* a hunger, a ravenous hunger, a wanting, waiting to be satiated. A longing and a yearning for...

A returning. A reclamation and remembering of your direct knowing.

The knowing, oracular and wise, that's instinctual and felt *through* your body. Your animal body.

Because these are the wildest of times and they're calling us to return to our wildest nature – to return to our 5,000+ years overdue, mother-loving true nature. Our source-ery.

And yes, it feels dangerous. They've had us fearing our own bodies, our power and magic for a l o o o n g time now. And yes, you feel exhausted and depleted. They've had us competing and at war with ourselves and each other for a l o o o n g time now. And yes, it feels dark, chaotic, unknown. They've had us scared of the dark, the chaotic, and the unknown for a l o o o n g time now.

And yet... you're here. And thank the bloody Goddess for THAT.

So, Source-ress, are you ready?

Ready to come to your senses, trust your instincts, and remember your magic?

Bring your attention back to the ground beneath your feet and then slowly work your way up your body, from your toes to the top of your head, giving each body part a li'l wink of recognition and love as you do so – you can touch it, tap it, stroke it. When you reach your head, take a deep inhale and on the exhale, give yourself a li'l devotional bow of recognition for being alive and present in these wildest of times.

You are the
Source-ress
of *your* experience.

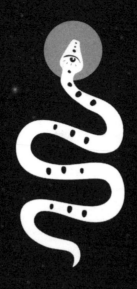

PART I

Come to Your Senses

*Hear your siren call, sing back
your wild, and reveal what's real.*

Underneath It All

What's underneath the masks that you wear, the labels you take (or are given), the gazillion versions of yourself that you've consciously and unconsciously curated and created to help you navigate and stay safe in a world where you feel you must perpetually prove your place and demonstrate your worth?

What's underneath THAT? Underneath the stories you've been told and sold? Underneath the societal programming? Underneath the need to simply survive and stay safe?

Look, there's NOTHING wrong with wanting to survive, to stay safe, and to enjoy other people's approval. It's just that for many of us, the norms of modern culture have drastically narrowed our innate ability to dream, create, and vision. Living in this digitized world with its constant screen time means our vision has literally been reduced to the size of a handheld piece of technology.

And our inability to see past that – to meet people in the eye; to be present (in order to be a fully seen and felt presence in the world); to really taste the food we eat; to feel the full range of our emotions; to trust our *own* knowing (versus the information we're bombarded with, which often has us choosing to pursue a societally approved way of living and experiencing life to avoid the risk of being called out, not fitting in, and being 'wrong'); and to gain perspective and practice discernment – has resulted in very few of us really knowing who we are underneath it all.

We're told, usually through a gorgeously curated social media account, to 'follow our wildness,' to 'run with the wolves,' that there's 'wisdom in our wildness' (and there IS, there REALLY is), and yet very few of us dare to ACTUALLY live our lives in that way. (Or would even know where to start.)

Reveal what's real

When I wrote *Witch*, I was very specific about my intentions for it. I didn't want readers to feel they had to *do* anything or *be* a certain way in order to 'wake the witch.' I simply wanted to provide them with guidance and support so they could find their own path, go on their own explorations, initiate themselves into their own power. Yet one of the key questions I received as feedback was, *I'm awake, now what?*

And that's a valid question in a world where we're under a h e a v y societal spell. In a world where we've been programmed to do as we're told, to override what we 'know,' and to do things the 'right' way (which usually means the way of the 'over-culture' – a term coined by Dr. Clarissa Pinkola Estes in 2015 to describe the dominant culture in a society, one that holds power over others), to doubt ourselves and instead to trust a reductionist, five-step, bullet-point plan for doing… well, just about everything.

Everything, that is, except how to connect with, and source, our supernatural, underneath-it-all, sensorial, instinctual intelligence. Our true nature. Our wildness.

You can't bullet-point your wildness. (Although I'm pretty sure that some people will continue to try.) In fact, trying to find the words to describe it here is proving really bloody tricky because words too are often a construct trying to make meaning of the ineffable.

**The feminine, and all that it is,
is not to be made sense of.
It's to be SENSED.**

It's not always possible to explain it intellectually and nor should we try. (Although, if it's not intellectually explainable, then under the current societal spell that would mean it's not real, valid, or of value, right? *Wink.*)

The good news is that your wildness *is* always available and accessible to you. It's IN your body. (But remember that the body, too, has been shaped by the over-culture – eat this, wear that, cut this, tuck that. We've been told what to think about it and what behaviors it can 'perform' – those that are lovable and acceptable versus those that are deemed slutty, unladylike, or simply NOT OK.)

We're told that embodiment – a felt sense and awareness of our body and its natural intelligence – is the way IN, and for the most part, it is. But BECAUSE the societal spell is *so* strong, many of us think that embodiment is *another* thing we need to consume, 'do,' and/or 'recruit' for it to 'work' and for us to be actually 'doing it.' Rather than letting our sensory system guide us there.

And it's VERY hard for us to trust our sensory system to guide us when we believe what we're told instead of believing what we sense and f e e e l. Because feeling the feelings... well, that doesn't always feel safe. Because feeling our feelings would mean trusting the natural intelligence of our bodies, and to many of us, 'natural' means wild, and wild has been sold to us as a loss of control, savage, uncivilized, and dangerous. So, for the most part, we're terrified of our body and its natural intelligence.

Let's take a deep breath, shall we?!

Live the questions

If we don't dare to get underneath all the acquired identities and labels, if we don't dare to know our real, wild, at-source self through the natural intelligence of our bodies (because we've been told and sold that it's too dangerous to trust ourselves and what lies beneath), how can we show up and live our life FULLY?

- How can we be fertile ground where strong roots can grow, and we become waaay more resilient to life's inevitable challenges?

- How can we have the capacity to hold the power and the parts of ourselves that we're calling back and reclaiming on our path to wholeness?

- How can we, as the author and poet Mary Oliver so beautifully expressed in her poem *Wild Geese*, 'let the soft animal of your body love what it loves'?

These questions are forever sitting in the center of my belly, and I invite you to let them sit at the center of yours, too, because we can't fully value what it means to show up and live a self-sourced life until we recognize all the ways we've been trained NOT to.

We can't reconnect with the body's natural intelligence without feeling and sensing it in response to the vibrational rhythm, magnetism, and frequency of Mumma Nature and the cosmos.

> We can't untangle and unravel ourselves from the societal spell and conditioning until we realize that we are NOT SEPARATE from life, we ARE life.

We're a part of a living, self-sourcing process that's bigger than us and yet intimately nourishes us so we can dream, vision, create, and innovate.

And THAT is how we begin to navigate a world that isn't set up in our favor: we turn our attention to creating a different one. We take the time required to dismantle the internal systems and structures that we've been told 'keep us safe,' so we can reconnect with what's real, with the natural intelligence of our bodies – our ancient-future wisdom and knowing – and trust ourselves as Source-resses to create from source, as source, an entirely new possibility.

Question ALL
that you've been
told and sold.

I Hear Her Calling

Like the author Anaïs Nin, I've often declared that 'I must be a mermaid... [because] I have no fear of depths and a great fear of shallow living.' Basically, I like to think of myself as the mermaid princess Ariel in the 1989 Disney movie *The Little Mermaid*. (Except, unlike Ariel, I don't often have an urge to be 'where the people are.' I'm a Scorpio and small talk is not and *never* will be my vibe!) Which is why, to get underneath all the stories that *I'd* been told and sold about myself, I turned to the sirens of the sea.

In European folklore, a mermaid (sometimes called a siren) is a part-female sea-dweller whose 'call' is alluring and seductive but ultimately perceived as harmful and/or dangerous to those who are attracted by it. Because succumbing to a mermaid/siren's song is ultimately succumbing to the wildness of Her.

This became all the more fascinating to my curious soul when I discovered, through one of my most favorite authors, Kathleen McGowan, that there's a reference to Mary Magdalene, the OG 'dangerous' woman, in *The Little Mermaid*. Yep, hidden among Ariel's underwater treasures is a depiction of the painting *Magdalene with the Smoking Flame* by the French artist Georges de la Tour.

Now, a lot of people have taken a guess at what this alludes to, but personally, I think it's a nod to the fact that like Magdalene, Ariel has been shackled by the over-culture and punished/reprimanded for her desire to have more.

There's something about Mary (Magdalene)

I first came into connection with Mary Magdalene (MM) through my connection with my own menstrual cycle. As I wrote my book *Code Red*, I went deeper, and I now have a lifelong heart-on for her. As a woman, as a consciousness, as a teacher, as an alchemist, as a portal IN to my own mistress-ry of the mysteries.

The deeper my connection with MM became, the more red-with-rage I became that for most of us, the menstrual cycle has been hidden and shame-laden (like so many other things that were put in the dark and called taboo – for example, sex, pleasure, money, feminine power). Because the truth of MM – keeper of the blood, sex, and magic mysteries, the 'scarlet' woman (when I create my own make-up range, I'm totally going to make a 'Magdalene red' nail polish and lip paint combo: *blood red*, obviously) – had been hidden and shame-laden too.

My anger and frustration were *her* anger and frustration. Because that's NOT the story we've been told. The early Christian Church stripped MM of her sacred priestess powers and instead depicted her as a 'prostitute' and a 'notorious sinner,' and in doing so, they stripped us *all* of our powers.

NOTE: I'm often asked for ways to connect with Mary Magdalene, to petition her, to pray to her, and for my personal interpretation of her. But ultimately – as with any/all of the goddesses, women, and mythos I talk about in this book – the most important thing is YOUR interpretation of her/them. YOUR relationship with her/them.

Beyond my own exploration and experience of MM, which has taken me *all* over the world, what I know with absolute certainty is that there's memory, transmission, and legacy always waiting for you when you enter into what author Sara Beak calls a 'red hot and holy' relationship with her.

Enter in, I dare you. I can't wait to hear about what you discover.

Can you hear *your* siren call?

So, if the Mary Magdalene portrait in *The Little Mermaid* is a nod to Ariel being punished for wanting to be more of who she *really* is (underneath it all) and daring to follow her own siren call, what if we're *all* ignoring/turning away from our siren call – our own song of alluring passion, pleasure, and joy – because we've been told that it's dangerous?

> **What if we've all been under the societal spell of conformity for so long that we don't know HOW to remember the power and magic that's held in the wild? OUR wildness?**

What if we could *all* access deep intel that's pre-nervous system, in the waterways of our own fluid body, which holds memories and wisdom that are waaay before fear and the unknown – which can/will/must be used to strengthen and to fortify us, *in* our human form, so that we can create and innovate. So that we can be of service in the here and now?

Look, like I say, I'm a Scorpio, and diving deep – literally and figuratively – is my THING. I've channeled this curiosity into my art: I've created a *SHE Sirens Oracle* in which I explore the siren call as feminine aspects of allure and seduction, pleasure, and purpose – a way-shower to our own freedom, agency, love, insight, wonder, and revealment.

Because let's be clear, the story of feminine repression is OLD. We can see and feel and witness its imprint in the jealousy, envy, and comparison we so often experience with each other. AND we can also see and feel and experience that the patriarchal, mechanized, industrialized systems and structures which have had us – women/sisters/humans – pitted against each other are crumbling.

Yes, the witch wound is very real AND we can also choose *not* to continue perpetuating it. Why fight the dying structures and systems when you have the capacity to create new ones?

What if... the siren call – the song that's been sung through the many layers of deep and primal oceanic truth held in your fluid body – is YOUR call, waiting, wanting, needing to be shared in the world?

Are you *ready*?

Hold the conch shell to your ear. Can you hear it?

Can you hear your oceanic siren call?

Calling you to be fearless in the pursuit of your Self Source-ery. To gather all you've learned and alchemized and metabolized from the exploration of your witch wounds. Calling you to respond by singing, at the top of your voice, *your* song – your purpose, magic, truth, medicine, and knowing – which will create the most incredibly powerful and potent birthing soundtrack for What Come Next.

FYI: Being 'ready' doesn't necessarily mean that it feels comfortable or easeful. It may do, but usually the very best miracles and magic and medicine are birthed in, and through, the chaos of times like these.

Yes, it's a big ask, but really, it's the ONLY ask. Because honestly, what else is there to do but reveal what's real, and to know ourselves so deliciously intimately IN our bodies? So that we become the most fecund and fertile landscape in which to create and birth into being an existence where we ALL get to thrive and flourish.

Every being has a song.

Every cell sings that song.

Our body is a divine symphony of electromagnetic frequencies.

Yes, you are SHE who IS a song.

SHE who can sing entire new worlds into being.

Our songs WILL all be different. AND they'll be completely in resonance with the frequency of Mumma Nature and the cosmos – our natural, wild intelligence.

INVITATION
SOURCE YOUR SOUNDS

You don't have to be a trained singer or anyone's version of 'good' to begin to sound and vocalize the song that wants to move through your body. Sonic vocal toning is one of my favorite medicines because it works with what's currently going on in your body to let your real and natural voice/song be expressed. What's produced by the voice during this practice can range from guttural, deep-in-the-belly sounds to cries, groans, and wails and sounds that seem ancient and not of this Earth. It's ALL possible.

* *My suggestion? Begin by putting a hand on your heart and a hand on your belly; then inhale and on the exhale, with your mouth closed, hum. Feel the resonance of the sound IN your body. Now see if you can move the hum to specific body parts. (Since the beginning of time, sounds have been used to vibrate and heal the body.)*

* *Practice this for a while – the act of humming is a great nervous-system soother – and then, as you begin to feel more confident about making vocal sounds, start to bring your attention down deep into your belly, into the space between your hips, and witness how source, life force, wants to be expressed through your voice. (Knowing that this can/will be different every time you do it.)*

✩   *Record the sounds you make with your voice and see if those you make in the morning are different to those made in the evening. Are the sounds different when the moon and/or your body is cycling through its phases? You're not judging whether it's good or bad - you're simply letting the tones, notes, and sounds of your song be revealed.*

...

You are a force. Of nature

Seas, rivers, baths, lakes – wherever there's water, I'm at my happiest and most free. Immersed, swimming, bathing, showering in it, I LOVE water. From a very early age, I'd declare to anyone who cared to listen: 'I'm from the ocean.' When I misbehaved, my grandpops would often threaten to throw me back there (and quite frankly, I didn't care, because I KNEW it was where I was from! Ha!)

And I was bloody right. Life on Earth began in the seas – every organism in our ecosystem responds to, and is biologically linked through, water. We live in the embryological fluid of our mumma's womb for nine months, so living in water is a core, cellular memory for us.

We carry the same mineral composition as seawater, too, which basically means we ARE all sirens who carry the sea IN us. We're from the sea, we *are* the sea. We carry the learnings and yearnings of our oceanic ancestors IN our bodies.

I'm blessed in that I currently live close to the sea, but when I'm away from it, I always carry with me, in my pocket or purse, what I call a hag stone. Different traditions call it different things but it's a stone with a hole worn right through it by the sea. In my lineage it's said that moving water protects us from negativity or from magic being used against us, so if we find a stone with a hole created by moving water, the stone holds the protection of the water and acts as a protective amulet.

Whenever I find a hag stone, I give a li'l nod to Mumma Nature for this hold-in-my-hand reminder that when we're in flow, we're a force of nature. A force capable of moving, shifting, transforming, and alchemizing things/beliefs/stories/experiences that we thought were literally set in stone.

Our underneath-it-all knowing

Now, if we're *from* the sea, if we *are* the sea, what if… and if you're into my Ariel and Magdalene analogy (whatta combination) you may want to dive into *this* theory/remembrance with me:

What if… a mermaid/siren is in fact a Source-ress who KNOWS:

The power and potency, magic and medicine, of her own wild waters?

That water is the source from which we came and the source that continues to flow through us?

That dwelling in the fluidity of our body is a perpetual state of creation, possibility, and becoming?

Because, although we may never have been 'in the wild,' there are things that the 'soft animal' of our body *does* know instinctually, and it's that underneath-it-all 'knowing' which is intuitive, sensorial, and oceanic and creates a longing – a deep, womb-like longing, a longing to return to something we cannot remember and have never experienced.

You KNOW that feeling, don't you? I KNOW you do. It's deeper than the socially acceptable desires that we've been told we're *allowed* to have and strive for. Yep, it's waaay deeper than that.

Look, we live in a world where computerization has occurred so rapidly that many of us haven't even noticed that our lived experience is out of sync with the rhythms of the Earth's electromagnetic field and the natural swirls, vortices, and pulses of its bodies of water. (Remembering that we too are bodies of water.)

So when (and I DO realize the irony of what I'm about to say, as I sit in front of a computer, tapping out the contents of my heart and belly) we sit still for long periods of time, or our system is bombarded by the continual buzz of technology and endless streams of information are coming in and at us ALL THE BLOODY TIME, it can be really hard for us to tune in, to experience our own frequency, to hear our unique siren call.

But we *do know* it. Yes, the societal spell has done a really solid job of separating and distancing us from what we truly want and desire, pushing us instead toward what *it* thinks we *should* want and need; and words like 'primal' and 'instinctive' and 'natural' are deemed 'untrustworthy' (especially in relationship to women); and our nervous system is continually being activated… AND yet (and thank the bloody Goddess for this), we *still* KNOW.

NOTE: Just to be clear – because there's a LOT of talk about how a 'dysregulated' nervous system is a 'bad' thing – there's *nothing* wrong with you if your nervous system becomes dysregulated. It does it to protect you, to keep you safe (and alive!)

It's just that many of us are in a perpetual loop of hustle, productivity, and 'must do' while teetering on the edge of overwhelm, anxiety, and burn-out, and our bodies are in a forever-state of activation that we simply cannot sustain. It makes us irrational, reactive, and judge-y, and our nervous system loses flexibility, capacity, and resilience. NOT OK.

✮ *Source-ery Support* ✮
Lemon balm

This easy-to-grow herb was one of my nanna's favorite cure-alls, and it's what I now refer to as my personal self-soother. Lemon balm is often called a 'herbal hug' because of its soothing effect on the nervous system. If you have trouble sleeping or need to return your body to a state of contented peace, you can use lemon balm essential oil in a diffuser or make a lemon balm tea – add fresh or dried leaves to boiling water and let them steep for 10 minutes before drinking.

(Honey is optional – although it's NOT in my world: I bloody LOVE honey and add it to EVERYTHING because it's the nectar of the Goddess. In fact, in ancient Greece, the beekeepers of the Temple of Artemis often planted lemon balm near their beehives to keep their sacred honeybees happy. Consider me a sacred honeybee!) NOTE: Lemon balm shouldn't be used during pregnancy or lactation.

...

Slow down and f e e e l

One of the main things I hear when working with women, specifically those on a spiritual path, is that for them, calling back their power, accessing their deeper 'knowing,' and what they then 'see' and 'feel' in response to that, can be WILDLY overwhelming to a nervous system that's often dysregulated. I get it – and this is *why* I'm sharing Self Source-ery.

Many of us are awake, but we're calling back our power to a body that's tired, not properly nourished, and burned out. We're following generically prescribed practices that we're told will help us to become 'more spiritual' – drink the green juice, wear the expensive leggings, eat the kale – yet for some, these actually create MORE overwhelm and MORE disconnect in the body.

When you're able to s l o o o w down, you're able to connect with your body; you're able to f e e e l your feelings, emotions, and sensations and find what works for you – what helps you to feel nourished, satiated, and sourced – so that you have the capacity to hold MORE…

More magic.

More joy.

More pleasure.

More vitality.

More creative force.

More source (power).

Now, many people, including me, find the act of sitting still and 'meditating' really bloody difficult (and in some cases, especially for those who have experienced trauma, sitting still with eyes closed can sometimes create *more* trauma in the system). It's why so many of us struggle with the concept of 'rest' and find it easier to 'get on' and 'keep busy.'

So, I urge you never to let anyone tell you there's only one 'right' way to do a thing, especially a 'spiritual' practice. If meditating in the conventional way, sitting still and paying attention to your breathing, doesn't feel good to you, don't do it. There are so many other ways to explore meditation; in fact, moving meditation (being mindful and aware of the feelings and sensations that occur as you move your body) can be way more useful (and feel safer) for those who have experienced trauma.

Also, I'm not saying DON'T meditate. Stillness is such a delicious gift to our system, but if being still feels uncomfortable to you and/or creates heightened anxiety, don't do it. At least not while it feels that way.

Finding a place of peace

A few years ago, I went on a silent retreat in Spain.

Ten days. Silence.

I loved it – once I got past the noise, resistance, and chatter that played on a repetitive loop in my head, obviously.

I remember saying at the time that if I wasn't married to a hot Viking, I'd stay forever.

I remember declaring that the peace was so profound that I met God there, and I loved on her. Hard.

I remember looking into whether there was any way to become a nun AND still have sex, because if there was, I'd definitely consider signing up.

I remember that combining the silence with darkness was a form of much-needed death training. I did it diligently. And later, I shared it with clients.

I also remember recognizing, in that place of peace, that the 'actual work' is being able to reside in that place of peace WITH the noise in your head, WITH the judgment, and WITH the overwhelm – not for it to be a place we escape to, or from.

But I forgot all of these things. Because someone who's at peace in, and with, their body and who they are – a person who's able to stay balanced in their center, their place of peace, when the world gets noisy and out of whack – is bloody powerful. So, obviously, it's not encouraged.

Sure, we can do a meditation class, or grab a 50-minute yoga session and wish the whole thing was that final 10 minutes spent lying in the *shavasana* resting pose (that's not *just* me, is it?) Or take a 22-day *Vipassana* (silent meditation retreat) or read a book about self-care and mindfulness. But REALLY being at peace with yourself and in your body is, I'd suggest, one of the most potent acts of deliciously defiant remembrance and reclamation of power.

Becoming sacred ground for YOUR magic

My system *wants* to remember. It wants to remember SO BAD.

Which is why I start with a daily commitment of five minutes of peace. *Not* meditating. Simply setting the intention to reside, momentarily, in a place of peace. In silence. In my body. Breathing. In for a count of four, hold breath for a count of three, out for a count of five. Drop down into the body and be there.

What we're looking to do here is become aware of our bodies and the full range of our feelings, sensations, and responses. Not so that we can try to 'fix' them, but so we can acknowledge them, learn from them, and then create practices and cultivate support that nourishes us; that allows us to get spiritually stretchy. (No pretzel shape-pulling is required. Unless you want to, obvz.)

When it became too gnarly for *me* to be IN my body – when I'd 'see' or 'hear' more than my system had the capacity to 'see' or 'hear' or 'feel' – I'd dissociate from my body. Yep, despite teaching yoga, movement, and embodiment for 10+ years, it wasn't until I trained as a somatic practitioner – until I immersed myself in the awareness of my own fluid body, got underneath all the stories, wounds, and trauma that I *thought* were who I was, and got curious about those 'what ifs' I shared earlier – that I realized it was here, in the life-giving fluid and flow of my body, that REAL embodiment, healing, and transformation can take place.

If I could slowly allow all that wanted to be present to come in and go out, like an ocean wave – so that, for example, my ability to 'see' became part of my lived experience – I could then create safety to 'see.' I could integrate my oracular and mystical visions into my lived and embodied experience IN my body.

Because, let's be honest, although numerous books and teachers encourage us to connect with our spiritual self, for the most part, for most of us – especially those who have chosen to join me here in this bubbling cauldron of Self Source-ery – it's navigating the lived experience of staying connected to our bodies and remembering our magic in the realness of the everyday that proves to be the most difficult thing.

It's why so many of us DO seek 'spiritual approval' outside ourselves. It's so much easier (in the short term) to do as we're told, instead of trying to develop intimacy with ourselves by s l o o o w i n g down and taking notice. (Of what's underneath it all.) Because underneath it all is where I found my *real* hunger was residing. An unsatiable hunger, an oceanic longing for what's real. For what's deep and organic, and well... *wild.*

I know THIS from personal experience too: to our thoroughly mundane self – the self that *is* navigating the day-to-day experience of life and living wild can feel... crazy. I've often asked myself: *What's wrong with me? Should I medicate? Should I get therapy? Do I need fixing?* (By the way, I've previously answered 'yes' to all of these and have had varying degrees of success, so there's NO judgment here.)

And I'm *definitely* not saying you should do it alone, either. That's how we got here – by NOT being in community, by NOT having the support and guidance we require to be IN our bodies and IN our power AT. THE. SAME. TIME. However, when choosing guides and communities, you *do* need to practice the fiercest discernment. Ultimately, you're looking for those who won't try to fix you but who will walk beside you and support you to find and to cultivate *your* own source-ery.

Return to source

I *have* dared to dive underneath it all, to connect with my fluid body, the knowing flow I spoke about earlier. That deep, deep longing and hunger for what's real is a need, a requirement, for each of us to realize and recognize that wildness is NOT the danger zone we've been led to believe it is – I know, shocking, right?

It's a return to source.

It's direct and real.

It's reconnection at source, to source, as source. As life force. An open invitation to follow goodness (not to be confused with 'good,' which, FYI, is a construct).

Goodness is what's underneath it *all*.

A glorious innocence.

Nourishment.

A knowing.

YOUR knowing.

And staying connected to source IN.YOUR.BODY – despite the inevitable cries of *you're crazy* or *you're spiritual bypassing* – is HOW you hear and connect and respond to *your* siren call. *Your* frequency.

Here's the deal though: you have to give yourself the time and space to get curious and to explore. As I've said, and will continue to say, there's NO five-point plan or formula, and if the idea of meditating or resting, or even taking time out to explore the practices offered in this book *does* create or heighten anxiety in you, this is an opportunity to get stretchy with *that*. As I explained, EVERY practice I share is an invitation, but *do* get curious about, question, and track what's going on for you if some feel more appealing than others – remember, self-knowledge is self-power.

INVITATION
STRETCHING YOUR CAPACITY

Explore moving from hyperaware reaction-and-survival mode into a more relaxed and stretchy rest-and-digest space where your body can breathe more deeply and where it's possible, even for a fleeting moment, to witness your body as a safe space for magic and source-ery to be present.

WHAT YOU'LL NEED

A candle; rose petals (optional); colored pencils and paper (optional); your journal and a pen.

WHAT TO DO

Surround yourself with rose petals or use a pointed finger to create an energetic circle of love and healing. Call in your spirit team – that can be ancestors, spirits, animal totems, or guides – in whatever way feels good for you.

✪ *Light your candle, declare your healing circle open, and either sitting or standing, place one hand on your heart and the other on your lower belly. Bring your attention to your breath. Intentional in-through-the-nose and out-through-the-mouth breaths. Do this for three minutes.*

✪ *Drop your hands but continue to breathe deeply and intentionally. Then begin to check in with your body. Use your inner sight to 'scan' your body, starting at your toes. When I say 'scan,' I'm asking you to trust yourself and your inner wisdom to let you know where there's pain or discomfort, numbness, sensations, or any energetic schisms in your body, and all you're doing as you scan is witnessing them.*

Really 'feel' each body part as you scan it. If you tend to disconnect from your body and struggle to 'feel,' gently touch and/or tap each body part as you scan it. Move slowly up your entire body, scanning each part internally and externally until you reach the top of your head. As you do so, keep track of any sensations, but don't judge them.

✭ *Next, bring your left hand to your heart and gently tap on your heart space. Really FEEL your hand making contact with the energy of your heart, and as you tap, tell yourself: 'I'm IN my body.'*

Don't think, f e e e l. Feel all the parts of your body that are touching a surface. Feel yourself IN your body. If you find yourself thinking, bring your attention to the sensation of your hand gently tapping your heart space, and allow the space you're tapping to respond.

✭ *Allow. Don't rush. If you don't feel anything, or it seems as if there's armor around your heart, tell your heart directly: 'Allow me to soften so I can experience more.'*

When you've started to soften, ask yourself, 'What is wanting/needing/ desiring to be sourced in, and through, my body?'

Look, this is a BIG question and one that will ultimately be a lifelong enquiry THROUGH your body.

So, don't rush it, and don't expect a fully formed response/guidance; in fact, this will rarely come as words, and for this reason, I keep coloring pens and paper to hand to try and 'catch' a mood or sensation. That's not always possible, either, and I've become really OK with that. You may have to learn to do the same.

When you receive a response/guidance, take notes (if you don't receive anything, ask that it's shown to you through signs and symbols that are made really clear to you in the next 24 hours. I'm not promising anything, but usually the more direct we are, the easier it is for SHE/universe/spirit to deliver). Remember that the ways you receive intel will be different, so let it ALL be present as you learn how it is for you.

It's here in your heart, in your body, that you'll discover your 'hell, yes' and your 'absolutely bloody not.' It's here that we hold the possibility of creating fierce boundaries and sticking to them. DON'T BE AFRAID OF THIS ENERGY. It's power. YOUR power. (Know that your mind will be super useful when it comes to implementation, but right now, stay in your body as much as you possibly can.)

★　*When you're ready to complete this practice, breathe in emerald-green light to the heart. As you breathe out, send golden-yellow light down and into the lower belly. Do this for three minutes and then declare out loud three times: 'I TRUST MYSELF. I TRUST MY BODY. I TRUST MY SOURCE-ERY.'*

★　*Thank your spirit team, blow out your candle, and close your circle.*

. . .

The hunger was
always the siren call
wanting,
waiting,
longing
to be heard.

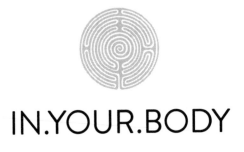

IN.YOUR.BODY

When you connect with your body, when you practice staying present to the feels and the sensations, you're able to build a relationship of safety IN.YOUR.BODY.

In many of my books (particularly *Love Your Lady Landscape*) I've spoken about the importance of connecting with the fulcrum of our power, the pelvic bowl (the bone bowl that sits at our center and supports and holds part of the digestive system, the bladder, and the sex organs). It's why EVERY morning I listen to music and move my body, specifically my hips and pelvis.

Coming into connection with your pelvic bowl is ALWAYS an invitation to come IN to your body and get curious. I consider it our in-built medicinal cauldron, a place and space of great power. It's our foundation – where we can connect deep to the root of Mumma Earth through the root of our own being and become sourced, at source, by source. Where we can alchemize, unravel, heal, reveal, and create (entire universes if we want to). And for me, it's where I create a real and true sense of safety IN my body.

As above, so below

So many of us hold pain and trauma (from this life and from past/future lives – ancestral, familial, AND cultural) in our pelvic bowl. It's why so many of us experience pain and dis-ease here; it's why so many of us feel unrooted, ungrounded, disconnected. Because if we're NOT in direct connection with our pelvic bowl, we're literally cut off at the root, disconnected from source.

**When our foundations are rooted and strong
in matter, we recognize that WE matter.**

Let's now come into what will hopefully be the start of a loving relationship with your potent and powerful cauldron of creation, by making circles and spirals and figures-of-eight – delicious symbols of the feminine – with our hips.

INVITATION
YOUR HIPS DON'T LIE

Through its direct connection with our throat and jaw – as above, so below – the pelvic bowl makes it safer for us to express ourselves and sing our siren song.

If you work at a desk or spend a lot of time driving a car, you may find that your hips and thighs become stiff and clunky. This can lead to energetic stuck-ness, dark and clotty blood at menstruation if you menstruate, and ongoing lower back pain and discomfort. Personally, I'd encourage you to do the following practice every day for the rest of your life, but for now, let's start with a little Shakira-style hip-sway love.

Honestly, you don't need instructions for this – there was a time when you naturally moved your hips to the rhythms of nature, the pulse of the universe, to the sound of your own vibrational frequency, so this is NOT something you need to learn.

✻ *Re-member. Tune in to your body. What music does she need today? Something fast and furious, or maybe something slow and sensual? My favorite hip-sway tunes are 'Shake It Off,' by Taylor Swift, 'Listen,' by Goddess*

Alchemy Project, and 'Cherry Bomb' by Joan Jett & the Blackhearts. You can either use these songs or make your own three-song playlist and then for 10 minutes... y'know, move your hips.

☆ *Circle your hips. Move them back and forward. Create figures-of-eight. Shake them. Tap them with your hands. The idea is to bring your attention to your hips, come into a relationship with them, and let them speak to you. For some of us, this will bring up emotions, as well as laughter and energy burps (or farts) – let it all be present.*

☆ *When your playlist is complete, put your hands on your hips (nope, I'm not asking you to do the 'Time Warp,' although you totally can if you want to!) and stand in complete stillness for a minute or two, letting the vibration of the movement you've created in your hip space continue to resonate from your center, out into your body.*

Your hips and pelvis create a magic cauldron within your body where alchemy is made, where you're able to turn ideas into manifestations, where you can create life, books, businesses, art – everything is possible when there's an energetic and physical flow of energy and vitality in this space.

· · ·

If we moved our hips more often and trusted the source-ery we hold within them, the world would be a whole lot more glorious. This I know for sure.

NOTE: If you DO hold deep trauma and/or experience pain and dis-ease in your hips, pelvic bowl, and/or womb if you have one, please seek support, either from me or another trained practitioner, as I know from personal experience that this can create profound changes to the lived experience.

It's a process

Our bodies are really bloody wise, and learning to listen to and feel the song and frequency that lies within and beneath is the MOST powerful spiritual practice. In fact, our flesh and blood carry the secrets and mysteries of the entire cosmos.

When we get underneath it all we KNOW. *You know we know,* don't you?

However, if you DO experience a dysregulated nervous system, it's ESSENTIAL to cultivate a relationship with, and expand the capacity of, your body to allow the fullest range of feelings and sensations and spiritual awareness to be present without overwhelm.

It's Self Source-ery.

It's how you care for, nourish, and nurture yourself so that you can stay present for longer.

It's how you tune in to the rhythm of your frequency.

It's how you tend to what it is that you truly long for. So that you get curious, and remain *ever* curious, about your deep oceanic longings.

It's how you feel less need to meet societal requirements and instead, become a walking, talking (often singing) invitation for society to meet you EXACTLY where you are, without bending and shaping yourself into something 'acceptable' and 'likeable.' (We're no longer here for that. In fact, those skills we use to shape ourselves into conformity are skills of our 'craft,' which, when used for Self Source-ery, can bend, shape, and create entirely new realities.)

It's how you, IN your body, become a nourishing and supportive container for growth and flourishing. A rooted-into-Mumma-Earth container that has the capacity to hold it all – magic and vitality and life force and creativity and magnetism. You know who you are (a mother-loving source *and* force).

> You know that your presence is your power, and that you're able to show up, take up space (unapologetically), act with fierce discernment AND be of service, without negating your own feelings and experience.

It's a process.

Ever-unfolding.

Not a goal to be finished or completed.

Yes, this is fortification, but not to protect or fight a broken system. It's fortification to create a deliciously stretchy capacity that creates space to experience and come into delicious and familiar relationship with it ALL – the magic, the gloriousness, the fire, the bliss, the pain, the devotion, the joy, the pleasure, the medicine. ALL. OF. IT.

YOU as a living ceremony to SHE

When I'm asked why I no longer teach yoga, I explain that it's not that I DON'T teach yoga, it's that I now share IN.YOUR.BODY.MENT® – whole body support and nourishment through movement, dance, breath work, and sound practices. Each class/session/workshop is curated to support participants in experiencing their body as a living ceremony to SHE – it's devotional and delicious, there's drum banging and sound making and foot stamping, and all the invitations and rituals I share in this book are forms of it.

What I've come to recognize – as a woman, as a human – is that our bodies speak truth. The pain, the tension, the numbness, the anxiety are all messages that add up to, 'Hello, shit is not OK in here.' Yet we've been taught, really bloody well, to either ignore, fix, or medicate the body. Rather than s l o o o w i n g down and learning to become literate in its cues, signals, and sensations, we do what we've been told to do in order to stay 'productive' and 'useful.'

This is definitely how it was for me, for SO long. When I'm asked *how* I became a woman who talks about vulvas and vaginas, menstrual cycles, power, and pleasure, I explain that it's because I was THAT woman. The woman who did NOT want to be IN her body. The woman who did NOT want to hear her body. I'd abandon myself at a moment's notice if it meant not having to f e e l.

Only, inevitably, if we don't listen to its whispers, the body *does* get loud. REALLY loud. Mine made herself known through endometriosis, polycystic ovary syndrome (PCOS), and pre-menstrual dysphoric disorder (PMDD) – yep, because I'd got really good at operating from the neck up, it got very LOUD 'down there.'

Actually, this is a good point in the book to respond to a question I'm asked *all* the time: 'Why *so much* 'down-there' talk? Am I less of a woman or witch without a uterus?' Look, I *do* talk about wombs a LOT. I celebrate the womb as a place of power, medicine, and magic because, as I mentioned in the opening to this book, doctors once threatened to remove mine and I've worked really bloody hard to heal her and love her and to recognize the power I hold there, and I want to support those who have had similar experiences to do the same.

I only ever speak, teach, and share from personal experience and wouldn't DARE try to be a spokesperson for EVERYONE. But of *course* you can be powerful, be a witch, be a woman, without a womb – abso-bloody-lutely.

FYI: You also NEVER need me, or anyone else for that matter, to tell you whether you're a witch, a woman, and/or a powerhouse of a human. ACTUAL FACTUAL.

Evoke your body remembrance

IN.YOUR.BODY.MENT is my personal call and response to anyone who wants to become literate in and wise to their own body's language. These practices were created to support, resource, and work in tune with the cyclical nature and rhythmic intelligence of *your* body.

Because when we do come in, come down, IN to our bodies, especially IN to our pelvic bowl, we can start to feel and experience our own rhythms, recognizing that like ALL of nature and creation we have a dance, a song, and a rhythm that's all our own. Like the ocean tides, we too ebb and flow, and we are MEANT to expand and contract.

So, IN.YOUR.BODY.MENT is an invitation to m o o o v e in a deliciously fluid, serpentine way with that rhythm (in that moment, knowing that in the next moment, it might, and often will, feel different).

It's this curiosity through moving our bodies, and the way we use our breath and make sounds, that evokes remembrance. At a cellular level. It evokes the wisdom held in the DNA of our being, in our mitochondria, which has been lying dormant, waiting to be activated, by us and through us. (In the same way that the Goddess, Ma, source power, has been ever-present for thousands of years, simply waiting for us to remember and activate Her, in us and through us.)

And when we can be WITH the feelings and felt sensations of the body through movement, breath, and sound we start to realize and recognize that we are in a dance WITH nature – that the water, the Earth, the fire and air, the moon and the planets ALL inform our lived experience. And that together, in that dance, we can co-regulate our nervous system, grow strong roots that support us to stay IN our bodies, and be more present and more coherent to all that's wishing to be seen, heard, felt, experienced, and lived.

The societal spell has us believing that everything is urgent. EVERYTHING. Our entire culture has been built on our ability to keep going. When we recognize and acknowledge that we're NOT machines that have been shaped and maintained to simply 'produce' – whether that's work (an olllllddd paradigm that stems from the Industrial Revolution), dinner, babies, sex – we can remember that we're wild and we KNOW.

We know how to restore.

To resource.

To transmute.

To shapeshift.

We return to a rhythm of life, to the ebb and flow.

We become someone who trusts their body, allows themselves to soften and to be in response to the invitations and gestures of life.

You, as a living process.

You are a living,
ever-transforming,
magical, and
magnetic process.

Walking the Labyrinth

My 'process' (*this* iteration of it, at least) began when my mumma died. The day after her funeral, I asked my husband, who I call the Viking, to take me to Chartres Cathedral in France. At the time, we were on the south coast of England, so getting to the town of Chartres meant an overnight ferry crossing followed by a two-hour drive.

Nowadays, the Viking is used to my siren calls, which are ultimately a need and a necessity to trust and follow my gut knowing and usually have us heading off on a wild and unknown adventure to a particular sacred site or locale somewhere in the world. Back then though, he was pretty unsure about what was *actually* happening. As was I, to a certain extent. But in the after-quake of death… what else is there to do?

So that's how, on a beautiful sunny morning in May, I came to be walking the labyrinth in Chartres Cathedral. (I now know that a LOT of the time the labyrinth, which is set into the floor of the central nave, is covered up by the chairs used for church services. Some suggest that these restrictions are intended to discourage people from discovering the spiritual power of this ancient 'walking the labyrinth' practice. All I know is that on the day we arrived, the chairs had been cleared, and the labyrinth revealed.)

The body of the Goddess

Chartres is a medieval cathedral that stands on what was once the sacred oak grove of the Carnutes, a Gallic (Celtic) tribe living in France during the Iron Age. They would come to the site to worship an image of a *Virgo paritura* – a 'virgin' about to give birth – in a grotto next to a sacred well. (So far, so sacred, right?!)

I walked the cathedral's labyrinth without reading about it beforehand or being aware of its cultural or spiritual significance, but ultimately, the same 'gut' feeling that had led me to Chartres, led me to the labyrinth. (It's said that the labyrinth represents the body of the Goddess, with a path defining its way directly into and out from Her center.)

Now, some enter a labyrinth with a question, a focused word, or an intention. Me? I entered with a broken heart, an emptiness where love used to live, and a longing. A deep, deep, in-my-belly-deep longing for Ma. Yes, for my own mother, the one who'd just died, but also the Ma that I wished to be. And deeper even than that, a longing for the BIG Ma. The Great Ma. The Ma who we've *all* been bereft of for 5,000+ years.

My gorgeous friend Hannah Hammond (@wayfaringlabyrinth on Instagram) is a trained labyrinth facilitator and she will tell you: 'You cannot walk a labyrinth wrong. You cannot lose your way, there is one way in and one way out. There is no need for fear in the labyrinth.'

Which is why an opportunity to walk the labyrinth is an opportunity to shed, like a serpent sheds it's skin, versions/stories/thoughts about yourself as you come to your own center and meet yourself there. (In the mystery.)

Come in, come down

When I reached the center of the Chartres labyrinth, I sat. Portal to portal, magnetic vortex to magnetic vortex. Now, at this point, the storyteller in me would love to tell you that something deeply spiritual, insightful, and profound happened here, but it didn't. There was literally nothing.

NO. THING.

I waited for what felt like hours (although in reality, it was probably only a few minutes), and I won't lie, I was a bit pissed off.

I'd come all this way for... well, NOTHING.

I was hoping for the kind of spiritual experience that others speak about. The Mary-like miracle. Some sort of Lourdes-style healing. In fact, if I'm honest, I wanted, more than anything, for SHE to invite me to curl up in Her lap, to have Her stroke my hair and whisper words of love into my soul and psyche while wrapping me in a nice warm blanket.

And when I met myself at the center of Her center, of course there was nothing but darkness, because that was exactly what was at my center – absolute dark nothingness.

I became aware that there were people waiting to enter the center of the labyrinth where I was sat, but before I got up, I instinctively put a hand on my heart and a hand just below my navel and dared to breathe deep into the darkness of that nothingness, to give my experience of absolutely bloody *nothing* a begrudging nod of reverence (because I'm nothing if not respectful).

And *that's* when I heard the words *come in, come down* IN my belly. (So much of what I/we hear is thoughts and stories in my/our head, but these words? They were spoken from my own belly and pelvic bowl.)

I waited a beat or two for more, but nope, that was it. *Come in, come down.* (Chances are, I may have even made *that* up, because *something* was better than *nothing*, right?) So, I got to my feet and started slowly weaving my way out from the center.

When I returned to the Viking, he presented me with a ticket. 'There's an underground crypt,' he said. 'They don't usually have tours but they're doing one in half an hour. Apparently, there's a well – I know you love a well – which is home to Notre-Dame-sous-Terre, Our Lady of the Underground.'

Come in, come down. So we went into the crypt, down into Her center.

Her center, my center

Although Chartres stands on the site of an ancient meeting place where all the druids in Gaul would gather annually in ceremony, it was pretty clear, pretty quickly, that the crypt tour guide wasn't big on the esoteric and was keeping things strictly VC (Very Catholic).

So, I nudged the Viking and asked him to go ahead and feign interest, ask questions – basically, to do whatever it took to keep the tour guide occupied – so I could hang back and have a little alone time with my center in Her center.

I said a li'l prayer at the crypt's well (where there's a well, there's source power, and it's said that at this site, there was once a rock in the shape of the vulva of the Mother Goddess – the *ultimate* source power), and then sat down beside a statue of Her: The Virgin Ma. Notre-Dame-sous-Terre, Our Lady of the Underground.

She reminded me of Sara-la-Kali, hailed as 'Queen of the Gypsies' by Traveller people the world over, whose statue is also underground, in the belly of the church in the village of Saintes-Maries-de-la-Mer in southern France. (My nanna had a picture of that statue of Sara-la-Kali by her front door and we all had to rub it for luck as we left the house.)

Now, while Our Lady of the Underground didn't invite me to curl up in her lap, or stroke my hair, or whisper words of love into my soul and psyche while wrapping me in a nice warm blanket (she's a statue), she *did* let me sit in silence with her, so I too could *come in and down*. INTO MY BODY. Into the depths of my own underworld.

I saw that many before me had petitioned the statue, but our tour guide wasn't keen for our group to do that. So, while the Viking kept her occupied, I pulled a pen out of my bag and on a page torn from my journal I wrote: *Our Lady of the Underground, this is my deepest from-the-belly truth…* Yep, I wrote Her a sneaky li'l love note from my center, cried a bit, and then snuck the note at Her center.

I didn't know it at the time (we rarely know any of these things at the time, do we?), but my mumma's death had set a new cycle in motion. I mean of course it had, how could it not? It was a cycle that would take me on the first of many labyrinth walks – real, metaphorical, and imaginal – and one where petitioning the statue of Notre-Dame-sous-Terre would begin what's now a lifelong dedication, devotion, and reverence to the Virgin Ma.

Known to me (and through me) as Source-ress.

Virgin Ma as Source-ress

Yep, to me, the Virgin Ma is the *ultimate* Source-ress. Wherever you find a Virgin Mother statue, dig a little deeper (come in, come down, remember?) and you'll often find that primordial source power was worshipped at the site *long* before a church was built on top of it. (In fact, you might just find that's *why* the church was built.)

To some, the Virgin Ma represents a mother and child – a notion for which I have a deep and loving respect – while for others, she represents what the French writer Jean Markale so beautifully articulates as 'the virgin giving birth ceaselessly to a world… in perpetual becoming.' SIGH.

As I wrote in my book *Witch*, contrary to what we've been led to believe, the word 'virgin' DOES NOT mean a girl/woman who hasn't had sex. In fact, a virgin is *a woman unto herself*, and her virginity is her *freedom*. The freedom that's found in her ability to self-source – to know herself through her cyclical nature, to initiate, to integrate, and to live fully with a courageously open heart (no matter how many times it gets broken) in the deepest knowledge and wisdom that all things inevitably die AND nothing ever really dies. Paradoxes, remember?!

In her book *Woman's Mysteries, Ancient and Modern*, writer and psychoanalyst Esther Harding said: 'The woman who is virgin, one-in-herself, does what she does – not because of any desire to please, not to be liked, or to be approved, even by herself; not because of any desire to gain power over another... but because what she does is true.'

So, when I speak of the Virgin Ma, I'm not speaking of her as a maternal mother, although she absolutely is/can/might be. I'm speaking of her as the very essence of Self Source-ery:

- **Virgin** (a free woman – independent, autonomous, untied)

- **Wholy** (a woman who is both whole AND holy)

- **A woman unto HerSelf** (a woman who knows herself, loves herself, tends herself, and celebrates herself)

- **Ma** who is perpetually cycling through the ebb and flow of creation. Who dreams, creates, and gives birth to herself, to the world, to the cosmos. Over and over again.

THIS is her mother-loving true nature. It's OUR mother-loving true nature.

SHE RIFF – WAIL YOUR WILDNESS

From the very first time I let out a cry from deep within my core, they have tried to soothe me, quieten me, pacify me, censor me, silence me.

My truest expression was to wail my wildness, and my wildness was silenced and denied.

It's a primal force, feared.

They've fed me and projected onto me
a diet of ideas and ideals.

How I should be.

What I should say.

How I should look.

They made it so that I no longer remembered
or recognized my wildness.

No longer knew which thoughts were mine.

Instead, I let their thoughts consume me whole,
and I wore them, like layers and layers of
uncomfortable skin that don't quite fit.

I wore them until it was so painful,
I could barely breathe.

I was suffocating.

So, I began to scratch at its surface.

I scratched so hard that the thoughts and
beliefs (none of which were mine) lay like the
dirt of the Earth beneath my fingernails.

I scratched so hard that I nearly reached bone. But
instead, underneath it all, what was revealed was me.

Vulnerable and bare.

Real and true.

Ready to wail my wildness.

Who am I here?

As someone who's bared her underbelly and talked about pussy
lips, vaginas, orgasms, menstruation, and women and their power in
the written form for more than a decade, AND who's traversing the

terrain of being a woman right alongside you, AND who, by nature, would much rather be sat under a duvet reading a romantic novel and eating cake than being seen and expressing herself out loud, in front of people, I'm not for one minute going to say that it's easy, it's comfortable, or even that's it's worth it.

Wailing your wildness, being seen, expressing yourself in a way that isn't always the most 'pleasing' to people, is NOT easy.

But what I do know is that it IS necessary. The HOW? Well, that's very much up to you. In fact, it's absolutely, categorically up to you. Take as much time as you need to drop, deconstruct, and even grieve for those layers of societal hypnosis, familial stories, and cultural programming. Go at *your* speed. Don't let anyone tell you YOUR truth.

Drop into your heart and then drop deeper into your core, into your belly, into your pelvic bowl – the most sacred container and cauldron of them all. Place a hand there if it helps and ask: **'Who am I HERE?'**

And keep asking until the voice that responds is YOURS.

Until the voice that responds runs clear and true through the waterways of *your* being.

NOTE: The artist Madonna, my forever-love, first crush, and first muse, holds and always will hold the frequency of Virgin Ma. In her 2016 *Billboard* award speech she shared that, 'I was called a whore. A witch. I was compared to Satan.'

I remember my mumma telling me off for singing the lyrics to 'Like a virgin' at the top of my voice when I was eight. (I wouldn't/ couldn't speak out loud when I was younger, but I would/could sing Madonna lyrics.)

I remember when I was older, friends sending me into a department store to buy a copy of Madonna's first book, *Sex*, because I was the only one 'brave' enough to do it. It wasn't bravery, though, it was pride. I was fiercely proud that a woman like her existed. A woman who was perpetually becoming. Who celebrated sex, challenged people, and didn't do as she was told.

Yes, I love Madonna's music – I can sing every word of every line of *The Immaculate Collection*. Yes, I love her for being skilled, sexual, talented, and outspoken. But mostly I love her, in all her spiky, cone-boobed glory, for being unapologetically HER.

NOTE ABOUT THE NOTE: While we're talking about unapologetic women, let's take a moment to love on artist (and one of the many women on my forever-love list) Frida Kahlo. I share this because one of my favorite artworks by FK, the somewhat gnarly *My Birth* – a piece which in her journals Frida claimed was/is a reference to her birthing herself – happens to take pride of place in Madonna's own art collection.

Don't you just love the way this SHE lineage weaves itself?

INVITATION
LOOK PAST WHAT YOU 'SEE'

So often when we look in the mirror, we only really see our reflection (and that's mostly to recognize what we've been told and sold is 'wrong' with us).

✶ *I invite you to stand naked in front of a mirror – ideally after a bath or shower, and with a big, compassionate heart – and really look at yourself.*

Can you do that? Can you do it without judgment?

Can you look past your body and 'see' what's there?

✶ *As you look at yourself, hear, feel, and sense any words, phrases, and labels that come up for you. Ask yourself which of these words and labels are yours, and then begin to recognize which were given to you by other people.*

Now tell yourself three times: 'I like, honor, and respect you.' (I use the word 'like' because it can be very difficult to start with 'love,' especially if your body has previously been a battleground and a place where you and others have called her names.)

★   *Stay a little longer. Place a hand on your heart, take a deep breath and declare out loud: 'I let go, with love, of all the names, labels, and identities that have kept me shackled to old ideas and paradigms of who I'm "supposed" to be.'*

★   *Now shake your body, let yourself make any sounds or noises of expression, and give yourself a big hug of love.*

...

This isn't a one-off exercise. You're going to have to do it a few times. (Social and familial conditioning runs DEEP.) You don't have to try and 'fix' any of it, but getting to know yourself in this way, stripping back the layers till you're bone deep (this WILL feel raw, but stay with it, there's gold in the discoveries you'll make), knowing what's yours to work with and what's been 'given' to you by society and cultural and familial conditioning, means that you can build foundations based on what's real IN your body.

Nothing comes as a surprise – you know ALL your parts and begin to own them. (You also recognize the projections of others and become much better at not accepting them as YOUR truth and experience.)

This creates wholeness. And a woman who's whole? She's a force.

Be a force. (Of nature.)

Wail your wildness.

Our Mother-Loving
True Nature

I won't lie, I've been known to use the word mother***ker a LOT in anger (*I know*, I have the mouth of a sailor). AND the raping and pillaging of Mumma Earth and Her resources – the disrespect and total disregard for our planet – DOES feel like/is a direct mirror of the way patriarchal, capitalist, over-culture systems and structures have/ are fucking us ALL, especially women and the feminine frequency and all it holds, so in most instances, I think my use of the word IS VALID.

But since my own mumma's death, and since meeting the Virgin Ma in the center of Chartres Cathedral – at source, *as* source – I've been on a Ma quest.

A returning.

To Her. To myself. To my center.

Taking the serpentine path, into the center of the wilderness of what it is to be motherless.

To that space at the center of each of us where we dare to dip into the numinous dark matter of NO thing and meet Her as a regenerative, self-actualizing force. Her as a 'curative.' Her as Source-ery. A place and space that has the capacity to hold power, to potentize it, and to birth 'perpetual becomings.'

The deeply powerful and potent magic and medicine that's found in the sacred act of being a *mother-lover*. (The very antithesis of a mother***ker.) A remembrance that a return to Her is a return to source. My/your/our own *mother-loving* true nature.

In delicious devotion to Mumma Earth

The disconnect between us, our bodies, nature, and the cyclical and rhythmic intelligence of all things makes it easy to forget how powerful and magic we are. We're part of an incredible biological and ecological system that's a delicious dance of connectivity. With our bodies. With the Earth. The seasons. The moon. The cosmos.

It's meeting the sun in the morning and feeling its rays on your face. It's bathing in the light of a full moon. It's sitting with your back to the oldest yew tree in the churchyard.

It's putting bare feet on the Earth, f e e e l i n g the underground presence of the mycelium network connecting every plant and tree in the forest.

It's bowing in deep reverence because that mycelium network can hear our song, read our energy, know our frequency, and it then shares that information with the entire bloody forest.

So, to really enter in, let your whole body soften and entangle itself in a deliciously romantic and devotional relationship with the Earth, with nature.

Your frequency, your siren song, resonating with Her frequency and Her siren song. SIGH.

INVITATION
LEAN BACK

As I'm writing this book – which, ultimately, is all the ways I can possibly think of to remind us ALL how to stay rooted, trust our bodies, and remember our own magic – instead of leaning in, I'm leaning back. Right back.

So many of us are forever leaning forward, looking into the small screen of a phone or a computer. Somatically, this activates our 'future thinking,' which means that we forward-trip and 'borrow' problems from the future to worry about, getting anxious about shit that hasn't even happened yet (well, at least not in THIS timeline).

But when we lean back, and I was taught this by Richard Strozzi-Heckler, founder of the Strozzi Institute, into our physical back, or even just allow our attention and weight to drop into the back of our bodies, we have the possibility and capability of accessing 3 billion years of wisdom, our ancestral self. The wisdom of your ancestors can be met if you settle back and trust your body and its wisdom. Their wisdom. Our wisdom.

I invite you to take a few minutes now to let your breath become deep and rhythmic, and settle back. You can lie on the floor or on a bed; you can lean on the back of your chair, on the grass, against a tree trunk – whatever you're called to. (I do this practice when I visit the Neolithic henge monument at Avebury in southwest England. Sitting against those ancient stones – so. much. wisdom.)

Now settle back into your back, the back of your shoulders, behind your spine and into the fascia of your back. Rest there and listen: **What do you hear?**

• • •

Courage (the mother-loving kind)

Now, to be the Source-ress – SHE who self-sources and is in a state of perpetual becoming – takes courage because, and I don't know if I've mentioned this, the societal spell is *strong*. In fact, These Times in which you/we currently find ourselves don't just call for courage, they call for *mother-loving courage*.

This is the kind of courage that involves you returning to the source of the matter. (Of the dark matter. Because YOU matter.) Trusting and loving hard on the Great Mumma and recognizing that YOU are a direct reflection of Her and all that she is.

Often, we become overwhelmed by our everyday experience of navigating a world that isn't made for cyclical and sensorial beings like us – one where war, greed, mistrust, and judgment are the dominant forces – so it's no surprise that we disassociate, check out, and/or become, consciously or not, a bit bloody cynical about it all.

It's why the hunger for our true nature, our mother-loving true nature, our longing for nourishment, often remains unsatiated. When we're perpetually stuck in a stress response, the body simply cannot prioritize nourishment because it doesn't feel safe enough to receive. Yet, as Source-ress, you recognize that we CAN unplug and detangle ourselves from the societal spell. (The one that wants us to be forever busy, overwhelmed, and stressed out.)

You recognize that you *always* have a choice. And when you choose to s l o o o w down, when you choose to f e e l, you begin to create the capacity to regulate your nervous system. And when there's enough capacity for regulation, your hunger cues can return. Yep, when we come out of a forever-state of survival, what's underneath it all is given space to reveal itself and our belly starts to growl for what it REALLY wants and needs.

SHE RIFF – REVOLUTIONS OF THE HEART

You are a force.

Powered by source.

In a world currently designed to 'trigger' and
'activate,' you – yes, you – DO give a fuck.
But you are VERY discerning about where,
and to whom, you give those fucks.

When you remember and recognize that you have your
feet planted firmly on Mumma Earth, that you're
rooted in the present, AND from that place you have
access to all that's been and all that's to come –
ancient-future – you can trust that you KNOW.

You know that rushing, judging, doing,
reacting is NOT what's required here.

Old tools from an old paradigm.

Take a beat. Take two or three.

S l o o o w down. Breathe. Receive.

Now… respond. Knowing that What Comes Next is imbued
with the magic and medicine of your direct knowing.

Because, as my forever-love the Sufi poet
Rumi said, 'Out beyond ideas of wrongdoing
and rightdoing, there is a field.'

I invite you to join me there. It's a field where
there's space for nuance. For opposing thought. For
multiple possibilities. All at the same time.

In a world that feeds us fear porn moment by moment,
to keep us in absolute 'them and us' thinking, it's
a courageous act not to judge and/or react.

To be generous with the capacity of your heart and
let it get stretchy with possibility. So that you
allow yourself to drop deep into your subterranean
landscape, get beneath it all, and 'see.'

To trust the clarity of your body knowing to
support you in responding accordingly.

THIS is an art

and it will start

ENTIRE revolutions direct from the heart.

Courageously choose love

We've been told that courage is what we need to 'fight' or be 'brave,' but I think courage is what we need to choose love. To choose to love and trust Her, Ma, source, amidst the pain, grief, suffering, anger, danger, fear, and intimidation, is to know what it is to love and trust *yourself* amidst the pain, grief, suffering, anger, danger, fear, and intimidation. The idea of 'choosing love' is often referred to as 'spiritual bypassing,' and I get that, especially if you're only ever paying lip service to it. But *courageously* choosing love is NOT passive. Far from it.

Obviously, it'll look different to each of us, but for me it's meant learning to trust myself and my body as my safe space. To trust that, despite getting really close to it at times, I'll no longer abandon or give up on myself. To trust that it's now safe to drop the protective armor and allow the belly growls of what's real, my true nature, to become the cues and clues for what it is I truly need, want, and desire so I no longer simply survive but thrive (and blossom and flourish).

> **Mother-loving courage is the big swinging ovaries of courage because it's cultivated through a deep love and trust in source.**

So, connection to source (while remembering and recognizing that you ARE source) creates solid and sacred roots. And if you feel rooted, you feel strong. And if you feel strong (and I don't necessarily mean muscle strong, I mean having the capacity to hold your potency, your magic, and your power), you trust yourself to make right and good decisions.

And if you trust yourself to make right and good decisions, you can show up to it all – life, relationships, and all that's tricky, painful, awkward, and fear-inducing (and delicious and pleasurable and juicy too) – sourced, with compassion and fierce, mother-loving courage.

Discernment and cunning

This is where REAL progress can happen. Because direct-from-source mother-loving courage isn't about being 'brave' or going into a situation blind – it's about loving yourself and trusting yourself enough to choose the right direction: for you, for your family/ community, for the collective. In THAT order. And well, that takes discernment.

Now, discernment is most definitely a practice for me, mainly because I'd always assumed that discernment was a 'fancy' way of someone trying to 'tame' my fire. I LIKE being fiery. I LIKE being able to express my rage – I'm really bloody good at it. I see and work with many women who have suppressed their anger for all the patriarchal/cultural/societal reasons and while I KNOW that it's an issue for some, it's not one that I've often experienced.

Kali Ma – goddess of time and cycles (and burning shit down and changing shit up: my unofficial title for her, given with ALL the love) and I have mud wrestled with our tongues out, wailing our wildness and anger and frustration to clear paths and catalyze change together for lifetimes, it seems. So, expressing my rage has NEVER been a problem. But containing it? Well, that has. Stopping it from hurting others? Yep, that's deffo been a problem too.

When people told me that my rage was out of control, I'd write in journal entries: *I AM feminine flow – don't you DARE try to tame me.* But what I KNOW now is that discernment is ALL about having a keen perception – it's a form of cunning.

Now *cunning* – yet another word that has negative connotations and is often used in a derogatory way to describe a woman who uses her 'feminine wiles' to override a mechanical/patriarchal situation – is actually rooted in Self Source-ery. A cunning woman was a woman who *knew* her feminine magic.

Cunning is KNOWING that you create fire and can burn shit down with it, but also KNOWING that if you hold that fire and use your body as a container to magnetize and amplify and bend and shape it, you're then able to use it with focus and clarity. Don't tame your fire – instead, harness it and use it with clear intention.

NOTE: I'm not saying that this is easy – and it's definitely NOT something I always get right. Which is why I call it a 'practice.'

INVITATION
CONTAIN, DON'T TAME

If you're currently experiencing a situation that's making you reactive, where there's a fire alive in you but you've no idea how to 'control' it, 'tame' it – in fact, fuck it, why should you tame it? You want to RAGE at the injustice of it all – I feel you.

I'm ALL about being our FULL expression. Yet I'm also becoming increasingly aware that although there are deffo times for Kali Ma rage – when the Tower card in the tarot is pulled and we burn it all to the ground – there are also times when we can hold the fire, we become the container for it, we potentize it, and we then choose its direction with intention.

✶ *Ask yourself: 'What is currently creating reactivity in me? Where in my body am I feeling it?'*

✮ *Now, take a breath. Hold it for a count of five, then release it long and audibly and ask that place and space in your body if it can hold it. If you can, let what you're currently experiencing be present IN your body without doing ANYTHING with it.*

✮ *Take in another breath, hold it for a count of five and then release again, long and audibly.*

Here, we're simply practicing holding the possibility of NOT reacting in our bodies, seeing if it's possible, and playing with how stretchy we can be.

...

Courage calls

We're currently living in a paradigm that holds us in a perpetual state of fear, one where everything has become a 'fight' or a 'battle' in need of a 'reaction.' One where we're told to put our attention on what separates us instead of what we have in common.

Generally speaking, that societal spell would have us give away and reject our own power, our instinctual, mother-loving true nature, to be accepted as the 'good girl.' It would have us ignore our underneath-it-all belly growls and instinctual knowing to be 'seen' as polite, to please and appease.

So, while it would be VERY easy to say and do what we're told is 'right,' and to react to everything that's unfolding right now in our world, both personally and collectively – all that's real and horrific AND all that's cloaked in illusionary smoke and mirrors – it's actually a fiercely courageous act to recognize the possibility and capability of the magic that's held in the power of *your* discernment.

• **What if the courageous thing to do** is pause, connect to source, trust, discern, and THEN respond?

- What if the courageous thing to do is create and love in the face of fear, pain, and anger, instead of fighting?

- What if the courageous thing to do is choose to love fiercely and cultivate compassion, instead of bringing each other down?

- What if the courageous thing to do is to trust ourselves? And instead of letting the fear, pain, anger consume us/silence us/lead us to react and retaliate, we pause, we source, we choose to tend to ourselves, our needs, our wants, and we love on ourselves. Not bypassing any responsibility, but first and foremost choosing ourselves, choosing love?

NOTE: You'll notice that here in our bubbling cauldron together, there are faaaar more questions than answers. Don't try to figure any of this out with your thinking mind. *Self Source-ery* is an invitation to feel and map *your* experience, *your* medicine, and *your* magic THROUGH your body. Yes, this is a book AND it's an in-real-time living enquiry and process.

🐍 YOU, self-sourced 🐍

YOU s l o o o w l y, with love and compassion, unravel and detangle yourself from the societal spell.

YOU remember your wild and hear your siren call.

YOU come into an intimate and lifelong relationship with your body and her innate wisdom.

YOU recognize and honor the power and potency of your pelvic bowl as an alchemical cauldron.

YOU cultivate courage (the mother-loving kind) to get underneath it all, to wail your wildness, sing your siren song, and return to your true nature.

Contain,
don't tame,
your fire!

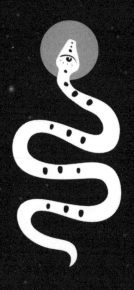

PART II

Trust Your Instincts

Return to the temple, reclaim
what you know, and set your
heart as your compass.

Take Me to the Temple

There was a time (you'll know it in your blood and bones too) when sacred temples dedicated to the feminine arts – ceremony, planetary observation, dance, song, chanting, rituals for death, birth, grief, sex, healing – were spaces and places to connect with and cultivate source power.

It's in the pursuit of revealing what's real and wild, returning to our bodies as sacred and fecund ground, that we activate a deep and instinctual temple remembrance IN our bodies. It'll be different for each of us, so as I share what *I* remember, let yourself soften to what YOU remember as we ALL return to the temple.

Beyond words

Since you're here, I'm sensing that, like me, you also feel that there aren't always words to fully express and explain a situation. What you're feeling and experiencing goes *beyond* words – they're sensations that may not even have names yet.

While this can be very hard for our 'I want to be a normal human' self to recognize as a power, ultimately that's what it is – a deeply feminine experience (all genders can access it, but I've found that it presents strongly in women) that's calling for us to trust our deepest body knowing and oracular nature.

Basically, if you find it very difficult to hold on to information and are more of a 'felt' experiencer – a reader of Mumma Earth and the 'energy field' versus someone who retains information from schooling and books – then this may be a skill/gift/bloody annoyance (depending on your current experience) that's already alive in you.

I used to plan and plan, producing reams of notes before going on stage or running a workshop; sometimes, I'd write the whole thing out word for word, only to get on stage, or sit in front of a circle of women, *feel* the energetics of those present, and be called to work with the energetic frequency of what was being felt and experienced rather than referring to my meticulously detailed notes.

Except, *trusting* what you feel and experience is bloody tricky if...

A. You don't know how to access and/or trust your body and its oracular voice and wisdom.

B. Like me, you tend to want to 'control' things. Paradoxically, this is ultimately why so many of us are *overly* controlling (well, unless you're a Virgo. *Wink*.) Because we desperately WANT to be seen as someone who can recite the 'right' dates or information and speak in soundbites on social media. And yet, well... we just bloody can't. (I even did a shit ton of training in public speaking and workshop planning so I could be THAT person, but well... I'm not.)

Past lives, this life

Back in the day, we'd have experienced a knowing that was beyond words, AND we'd have known how to access words and songs and incantations (our siren call, our tones, our notes, our healing frequencies) to bend and shape and create reality. And as I share that, you'll probably remember...

Memories of times when you'd sing over water and watch its shape and form shift and dance before you. When you'd speak and sing entire realities into existence with your words while in communion with source. When members of your community would come to you for the oracular wisdom you spoke directly from deep in the cauldron of your belly and pelvic bowl.

And I bet that, pretty soon afterward, you'll also remember why you might *not* be so quick to do that in *this* lifetime. I was mute for many years of my childhood – I didn't dare to speak. I know now that there have been lifetimes where I've had my tongue cut from me and where my jaw was smashed with an axe because I was speaking my magic and medicine.

And there's a chance that somewhere, throughout the lifetimes and timelines that *you've* experienced, you too may have been punished for speaking and singing in that way, and from *that* place. Maybe you've been spoken over, condescended to, shushed, called names, trolled/canceled online, or silenced (verbally, psychologically, or physically). And you too have felt the fear: the fear that it's 'not safe' for us to speak/write/share/sing our original truth song – which is ultimately our medicine to the world.

You/I/we live in a culture that really benefits from us NOT hearing/listening to/trusting OUR siren call. Because if you/I/we DID have the mother-loving courage to trust, and then to speak/sing/live OUR truth, it would ALL fall apart. ALL. OF. IT. The patriarchal constructs and systems that try desperately to keep us asleep/docile/tame/compliant would ALL fall apart.

Yet deconstructing all that's…fucked is a REALLY hard ask for our 'good girl' conditioning. We've been told that we're 'safe' within those constructs and systems; we've been told that we 'belong' within them. Yet is anything ever *safe* if it doesn't allow us to be curious and to express what feels real and true for us in any given moment (and also to be really OK with us when we change our mind?)

It's why I think it's SO important for all of us to have access to spaces, circles, and containers that support us in figuring out and working through our thoughts and feelings and expression without being judged or called out or explained to. I created the SHE Power Collective for this VERY reason (it's an online community that you're very welcome to join: www.thesassyshe.com/shepowercollective).

Forever in process

We're *in* process, and that process doesn't always have to be a meme or a 'teaching,' but it *does* have to be honored.

Why? So that we can become fortified.

So that we can remember. (Y'know, the stuff we knew before we forgot.)

BP (Before Patriarchy).

When we were oracles.

When we trusted ourselves.

When we trusted our wisdom.

When we trusted our power.

When we weren't made to feel small, inadequate, or less-than for having a voice and opinions.

When we didn't have to keep second-guessing ourselves or worry about what other people thought of us.

When we supported each other and held space for each other's experiences.

When we were unapologetic truth tellers.

> What the world wants and needs – and
> damn it, what *I* want and need – is for us
> to share our stories, our medicine, and our
> ever-revealing 'real' (our whole, raw, vulnerable,
> messy, glorious in-the-moment truth).

Not the so-called 'truth' of the 'good girl,' who says what she 'thinks' others want her to say so that she'll be liked and accepted. Not an over-rehearsed speech with carefully planned soundbites. Not a carbon copy of someone else's truth. How it is for YOU. In THAT moment.

YOU get to choose how you use and share your voice. (In fact, YOU get to choose how you use and share your art, your fullness, your anger, your quiet, your stillness, and your joy too.) For Goddess' sake, please don't let anyone tell you HOW to show up. Let how it is for YOU – your own truth, your own voice – lead your agency.

JOURNAL PROMPT

How does the idea of speaking your ever-revealing 'real' f e e l for you?

Does it feel scary to speak and express your truth? Do you know what your truth currently is? (It's really OK if you don't – that's why we have this space together, in this cauldron of possibility, to explore and experiment within.)

The curse of Cassandra

For some of you, speaking the true-to-you truth, singing *your* song, might feel like the curse of Cassandra. Do you know that ancient Greek myth? Cassandra, it's said, was a flame-haired beauty and a daughter of the king of Troy, so it made total sense that the god

Apollo wanted to romance her. He crushed on her HARD. So much so that in a bid to 'woo' her, he 'granted' her the gift of prophecy.

However, what many of the PG versions of this tale fail to share is that in return, your man Apollo wanted sexual favors. What they also fail to share is that Cassandra – a Source-ress, one of us – was not a woman who simply did as she was told, and she declined his advances.

Apollo got angry and turned the gift of prophecy that he'd 'given' Cassandra into a curse. One that meant she could see and foretell EVERYTHING, but no one would believe her. (My personal interpretation of the story? Cassandra was already a powerful prophetess and *that's* why Apollo was attracted to her. She didn't want to make out with him, so in true ouch-my-ego-got-crushed revenge, he devised a PR campaign throughout the land to prophecy-shame her, turning her gift into a 'curse' by ensuring that no one believed her.)

And it worked, because throughout time, Cassandra's been described as 'crazy' for the things that she shared; in fact, almost all the ancient Greek myths that refer to her say that she was 'insane.' Which is why it will come as NO surprise that, even now, in this time and space, if and when we choose to share *our* voice and magic, we too are often called 'crazy.'

Our natural skills, gifts, and talents – to feel, to sense, to see, to experience the subtleties of energies, to alchemize in our bodies our innate magic – are often pushed aside and called 'fantasy' or made-up. So, is it any wonder that we don't dare to trust ourselves, our bodies, and our magic? That you don't dare to anchor into the center of your truth, your own wisdom, your own medicine?

In a world where we've been taught that someone else ALWAYS knows better/more than us, choosing NOT to outsource our power, magic, and medicine can be hard/really uncomfortable.

When I witness a woman's rage being 'soothed' because it's deemed 'too much' and a bit 'spill-y' (totally a word), or her instincts being ignored or overridden, or her being told what she needs to do, be, wear in order to fit in…

I just want our temple back.

So that we can gather and be supported in embracing our bodies and our magic as a glorious ceremonial landscape that's acknowledged, respected, and fucking revered. Is that too much to bloody ask?!!!

You are forever
in process
(and progress).

Meet the Pythoness

My return to the temple began when I heeded the call to come in and come down. I invite you to do the same. Come in, come down, to the center of *your* truth, wisdom, and magic and meet the pythoness.

Now, it will come as NO surprise that the word *pythoness* was once used – and not in a good way – to describe a woman who spoke from the bottom of her belly. A feat which Joseph Glanvill, a 17th-century writer, philosopher, and clergyman, declared was 'as strange as anything in witchcraft.'

Of *course* he did.

Reclaim your center

And, as with every word that's ever been used against us, the word pythoness holds power. So, the invitation, *my* invitation, is to reclaim it and in doing so, to come in, come down. Reclaim your center, your belly, your pelvic bowl, your knowing, your voice, your ability to 'see' what you speak and then create it.

The pythoness is the voice that resides deep down in your belly. Coiled in your pelvic bowl, she's a primordial, creative force, a power source that's generating the whole bloody planet and is held in YOUR center.

She's real *and* she's mythos. And she *knows*. She knows ALL. THE. THINGS. It's gnosis. Although the Greek term *gnosis*, or knowledge of spiritual truths, is often linked to early Christian teachings, it's WAY more than that – it's visceral, deep, and divine mystical knowing. It's (g)knowing.

She is Lilith (known to some as Adam's 'disobedient' first wife, who was banished from the Garden of Eden because she refused to be 'subservient'; known to others as a 'demonic' folkloric figure; known to ME as fierce and really bloody powerful).

She who knows that NOT following her longings and instincts would literally destroy her magic, her own fruits within, the fruits of Mumma Earth. Far from being the serpent of 'deception' and 'temptation,' as we've been led to believe, she's untamed and unapologetic. She's wisdom and liberation.

Now, Lilith has had her fair share of defamation, although Cassandra, Mary Magdalene, Hekate (the Greek goddess of darkness and witchcraft), and Madonna are DEFFO up there with her in the Sisterhood of the Maligned (is that not THE best name for a girl band?), and she *knows* the mother-loving courage and self-responsibility that's required to choose.

And it's *always* a choice, to defy the stories we've been told (the ones that have been around for … oh, I don't know, 5,000+ years). Because honestly, they're getting really bloody boring now. Stories like…

Of *course* you can have a voice – although you must say things that are agreeable and compliant.

Of *course* you can have a voice – but make your words palatable and inoffensive.

Of *course* you can have a voice – but don't be TOO powerful or TOO much, yeah?

Do you dare to bite the apple?

The pythoness wants you/me/us to bite the apple, to devour the apple, to savor and get as much bloody pleasure as we can from the apple, so that we DO have the mother-loving courage to choose our own knowing – our innate wisdom and magic – over the illusion of 'good,' 'perfection,' and 'conformity.'

Do you dare to bite it? The forbidden fruit from the tree of knowledge that was offered to Eve by the serpent (who, in my favorite telling of the biblical story, was actually Lilith) in the Garden of Eden? In the fairy tale *Snow White* the apple is the 'poisoned' fruit that the queen makes Snow White take a bite from. And when you cut an apple across its middle, it reveals a five-pointed pentagram, the shape that the planet Venus makes in the sky across her eight-year cycle. Forget what you've been told – the apple is an initiatory portal IN to the feminine mysteries.

∿ RITUAL: CONNECT WITH THE PYTHONESS ∿

Make yourself comfy beneath the light of a full moon (you can do this practice anytime, but a full moon will ALWAYS add a little extra witch drama to the occasion), ideally sitting upright with the soles of your feet connected to Mumma Earth.

WHAT YOU'LL NEED

An apple.

WHAT TO DO

Evoke *your* pythoness by devouring the apple with eight slow, defiant, and intentional bites.

✶ With each bite, connect with and meet yourself. Then set an intention at each of your chakras:

Crown – 'I ask for your support to know myself and my authority as Source-ress, as self-proclaimed queen.'

Throat – 'I ask for your support to know myself and to speak my truth.'

Heart – 'I ask for your support to know myself and to trust my heart and its capacity to love.'

Solar plexus – 'I ask for your support to know myself and to trust my power.'

Sacral – 'I ask for your support to know myself and to allow pleasure and eros to be ever-present.'

Root – I ask for your support to know myself and to know that here in my body, no matter what's going on in the world, I'm my own safe and sacred space.'

Come in, come down.

✶ After the eighth bite, inhale, hold your breath, and on the exhale, make a long, snake-like sound: 'sssssssss.' (Back in the temple days, the priestesses of the goddess Isis – the great Egyptian mother goddess who represents healing, fertility, and magic – would repeat her name, over and over, emphasizing the last syllable like the hissing sound of a snake, the sacred sound of Ma. The sound of Self Source-ery.)

Let the sssssssss sound meet the full exhalation of your breath, all the way to the pause-point at the end of the exhale, and then repeat. Do this three times or 13 times (and know that how it sounds and feels, its intensity and what it evokes, will vary depending on where you are, the time of day, the moon phase, and current feels).

✴ Next, come to your feet *or* stay seated (your call) and gently move your hips. If it helps, place a hand on each hip and s l o o o o w l y and gently undulate and rotate – make loops, make figures-of-eight, stir your cauldron. Create movement in your pelvic bowl, in your entire fluid body. Don't use your hands to guide your hips, though: they're there simply so you have awareness of your body. Then slowly let the pythoness awaken in you and move YOU.

You can do this for as long as it feels good and juicy in your body, but I'd suggest around five to nine minutes, before sitting or lying down and allowing there to be a delicious pause. As you rest, bring awareness to your feelings and sensations. There's nothing to DO, and you're not looking to 'fix' anything – you're simply witnessing, allowing yourself to be curious. To receive, listen, feel, and breathe. Let your body speak, while you listen.

• • •

It's in this practice and process that, much like the serpent, you're both relaxed AND aware. You can digest and integrate the sensations and energies (while also letting go of what you don't need) and feel safer to drop deeper into your body, deeper into your knowing and deeper into your prophetic pythoness knowing. The deeper you drop into your body and its sensations, the easier it is to *know* your truth.

~ RITUAL: BELLY TRUTH RIFFING ~

The previous ritual may be enough to awaken your pythoness. YOU are creating the relationship with the pythoness in YOU, so trust yourself. If you're called, though, you may want to dive a little deeper and do some belly truth riffing with her.

WHAT YOU'LL NEED

Your journal and a pen; colored pencils and paper (optional).

WHAT TO DO

✱ In your journal, write the following words: **This is my deepest, from-the-belly truth.**

Now, close your eyes, place your non-writing hand below your navel, and breathe IN to the space that lies beneath the palm of your hand, between your hips, your cauldron, and into your pelvic bowl.

Imagine the pythoness coiled at the core of your being. Imagine that you KNOW she's primordial power, creativity, and wisdom. Coiled in the center of YOUR being.

✱ Welcome in the pythoness. Let her know that you'd like to work with *her*, the oracular voice of the underground serpent. Of Lilith. Of deep knowing, NOT information and facts, and write and express from THAT space.

If writing isn't your thing, record any sounds, songs, or phrases that want to move through you. If you play an instrument, make sounds that are evoked through what it is you're experiencing. Sometimes it's easier to simply make marks on paper, using colored pencils, in response to HOW the pythoness makes you feel.

· · ·

Every time I sat down to write *Self Source-ery*, I'd move my hips and do a few rounds of 'sssssssss' breaths to connect with *my* pythoness. I'd ask: 'Am I speaking my deepest, from-the-belly truth? More importantly, do I, and can I, trust it?' I'd do this to make sure the place I was speaking/writing/sharing from was my primordial, instinctual, divine inner authority. That I was sourced, at source, by source.

Take it s l o o o w l y. If the pythoness in *you* has been ignored, numbed, or not heard for a while, if at all, she may need a li'l coaxing and encouraging. So be gentle, with her, and with yourself, in the process.

The cyclical pythoness

The pythoness is our reminder that dwelling in our oceanic yearnings, the wilds of our perpetual becoming, won't always feel safe. As we ALL navigate this time-between-times, personally and collectively, nothing is certain. **NOTHING.**

It's uncomfortable. And it makes us vulnerable too, doesn't it? For me, it feels like I've accidentally posted a story on social media with me baring my boobs and I can't find the delete button. (I've never done that, BTW, but clearly, it's playing on my mind. Ha!)

You need REALLY strong roots in order to stay stable in this place and space, and even then, no matter how stretchy your capacity is, an innocent comment from someone you love can *still* knock you sideways.

I find this WAY easier to deal with in my pre-ovulation phase – when my skin is thicker, my tongue isn't so sharp, and my ability to see the light in situations is MUCH more heightened. And yet, it's in the second half of my cycle, my pre-menstrual and menstrual phases, that I've really learned to meet the pythoness IN the uncertainty and not knowing and to work WITH her as an ally.

NOTE: Personally, I think this is why the perimenopause and menopause have been packaged and sold to us as the time when women are no longer 'useful' to society – when in fact, the very opposite is true.

If the menstruating years are when we learn and experience a glorious death-and-rebirth practice each and every cycle IN our bodies – when we move through *all* the phases and seasons of womanhood every month – when we stop bleeding, it's because we no longer NEED to bleed; we no longer need to initiate into power because we ARE power. Every cycle of our bleeding years is initiatory, taking us deeper and deeper into our own living mythos.

The pythoness won't create safety – no, that's not her thing AT ALL. But she *will* compel you to relax into your being, to breathe fully, and be present in that time, space, and moment, so that you can be in collaboration with what's life-giving and in alignment for YOU. So that you're able to trust *yourself* as safe space.

THAT is Self Source-ery.

✫ Source-ery Support ✫ Prophetic pythoness

When I can't understand why I've 'forgotten,' why I've slipped back into old habits, conditioning, and stories *again*, I create this essential oil blend for my diffuser before I go to bed. It helps me to use my dream time to remember that I know what I know.

Add four drops of neroli, four drops of jasmine, and five drops of sandalwood to water. Neroli and jasmine are both dreamwork oils, and sandalwood allows us to work with the subconscious: the serpentine energy that's undulating and weaving through your psyche.

• • •

Affirm your (g)knowing

I sometimes think that I eat what I call 'noisy food' – things that are high in sugar and have very few nutrients – so I *don't* have to hear the truth, Her truth, *my* truth. And if this is the case for you, too, remember to start s l o o o w l y.

Build a relationship of 'like' with what you (g)know. It takes time and practice and a metric shit ton of care and compassion, but every time you experience it, affirm it. Place a hand on your belly/pelvic bowl, give it a rub and say: 'I trust you.'

Yep, for me, in the not-knowing, in times of uncertainty, in the most uncomfy of places and spaces, the pythoness has become a beautiful remembrance and support that up-levels *my* ability to trust myself and *my* body wisdom. In fact, the uncertain time-between-times becomes a daily practice ground in self-trust.

Trusting that it's a pussy-deep truth that I no longer need an intermediary between me and source because I KNOW. (*Psst! So do you.*)

Trusting that my intuition, gut feeling, tingles, and goosebumps are all signs that I KNOW. (*Psst! So do you.*)

Trusting that in this time-between-times, in this space of not knowing, I'm a total paradox, and still I KNOW. (*Psst! So do you.*)

SHE RIFF – I REMEMBER

I remember.

I remember that I'm bloody glorious.

I remember that I express all that I am on
both the inside and out, without apology.

I don't fear the opinions, judgment, or thoughts
of others as they're simply projections.

I don't explain myself to others. Instead,
I create and express and share.

Unbound.

Forever unbound.

I have no time or place to hide my light or play small.

I remember.

I call back all my rites, wisdom, and
templates from ALL the timelines.

I know what it is I need to flourish and feel nourished.

I ask for it, I seek it out, I don't settle for
less than what I know I need and require.

Diva? Possibly.

Devi? Absolutely.

Real AND mythos

Over time, meeting the pythoness *may* have you asking yourself: *Is it me? Am I primordial Earth wisdom? Am I source power?* Yes, you are, and sometimes that's FAR too big a concept for us to get our thoroughly human heads around. Which is why the pythoness is representational, archetypal, deeply mythological, AND very *real. Wink.*

But it would serve no system or structure that currently exists for us to remember THAT. It's *why* we're remembering how to self-source. So that we're sourced, at source, with the power and creativity and magic and medicine, the stretchy capacity required to hold it and to potentize it in order to create and birth entirely new ways of being. It's why I can't see any option other than for you/me/us to practice trust.

Trust that your (g)knowing – your instinctual wisdom, which has been deemed 'primal,' 'dangerous,' and 'feral' – is intel about your mother-loving true nature.

Trust, witness, and recognize that the second half of the menstrual cycle (the pre-menstrual and menstrual phases) and the second half of womanhood (perimenopause and menopause) are NOT the 'barren wastelands' we've been told and sold they are, but potentially delicious playgrounds for us to 'come to our senses' and rewild ourselves.

Trust your relationship with the pythoness as both real and mythos – allowing what's imagined in your very real dreamtime to coexist as a reality in your human body.

So, you can detangle yourself from the distractions and distortions of the societal spell/stories/conditioning that have had you believing that you and your body are broken, wrong, and untrustworthy and instead, begin to believe and trust that what you see and receive and feel as wisdom, inner sight, and intel *through* your body is YOU, self-sourcing.

I've NO doubt that the fact you're here in the world right now, that you're in this bubbling cauldron of exploration, is because you *see* and because you *know*.

SHE RIFF – YOU KNOW YOU KNOW

You may have noticed a stirring deep within the core
of your being, a cosmic wink, a twitch, a nudge.

A call within.

To listen.

To your deep knowing.

A knowing that looking outside
yourself no longer serves you.

A knowing that looking outside yourself is no longer an option for someone who's awake.

A knowing that what really matters, what's vital, is to look within. Because you KNOW.

The Queen of SHEba, Isis, Mary Magdalene, Lilith, Sophia, Eve — they all knew.

And now, you know that you know too.

This isn't a riddle, it's a remembrance.

It may not look how you expected it to but knowing doesn't LOOK like anything.

Be open to the awesomeness that's about to occur as you remember what you know IN.YOUR.BODY.

Watch as negative thoughts are replaced by powerful, supportive ones; feel as doors start to open for you; be aware that you're being asked to step up and speak up. You've got this.

You don't need to research, be better, or do more.

Trust yourself.

Start taking actions that reflect the wisdom of your heart, gut, and pelvic bowl.

Be of service and treat yourself and others with the kindness and compassion of someone who KNOWS who they are.

Bite the apple.
(I dare you.)

All-Seeing

My connection to the pythoness within *me* has strengthened my trust in what I'm able to 'see.' I come from a Traveller family (my nanna was an Irish Traveller and my dad's family were Romani), and all the women in my matrilineal line had what was called 'the sight.'

Now, 'the sight' isn't something that's possessed *only* by women in Traveller communities – I believe we ALL have access to it – it's just that in my family, it was cultivated. My mumma chose to 'ignore' hers, though, and refused to share much of what she 'knew' with me. But luckily, I spent a lot of time with my nanna, so I got old-schooled in it and was told, in no uncertain terms, 'You're not to tell ya mumma.'

So, does having access to 'the sight' mean I'm immune to fuck-ups because I can see what's unfolding? NO. Does it mean I can see how everything's going to end? NO. Does it mean I can figure out the lotto numbers? I bloody wish.

I'm human and part of my experience here at Earth School is to experience the human-ness of it ALL. But what this 'all-seeing' aspect *does* offer – when I get out of my own way, that is (and THAT'S a daily bloody practice for me) – is a deep and clear connection to the wisdom, clarity, and discernment that reside within me. So, when I take a breath, create some space, and come in, come down, I can see EXACTLY what's going on.

If someone's angry and they're aiming that anger toward me, I'm able to see all the parts that are in play IN THE MOMENT. I can see my part in it – maybe I've pressed a button; maybe I'm just in the wrong place at the wrong time and I'm taking the brunt of their anger. Or maybe – and I can't POSSIBLY believe that this could be true – I've messed up and/or done something wrong. I *know*, I doubt that too. Ahem.

But also, I'm able to see *why* that person's lashing out, and *where* their fear and pain lie. If it's someone who menstruates, I can 'usually' tell where they're at in their cycle. And of course, I have access to moon placements and cosmic alignments too.

Inner tuition

This inner sight is inner tuition – internal wisdom and schooling that enables me to respond and *not* react. I can assess and discern situations, making sure my heart, belly, and pelvic bowl are in total vibrational alignment with the decisions I take and the choices I make.

This supports me to ground, root, and center my energetic frequency so that I show up accordingly because I trust what I SEE, FEEL, and KNOW. I can 'see' what's going on. I can read between the words that are spoken and I can hear what's *not* being said. I know when I'm being lied to AND I know when I meet real.

For me, this inner sight is at its strongest (and most useful) during my pre-menstrual phase (if you menstruate too, it might be worth noticing where you're at in your cycle as you read this). The place where my inner critic was once at her loudest is now the place where I see everything AS IT IS (I mean, she still hangs out there but she's no longer the loudest voice). No gloss. No fancy filters.

People who I 'might' have compared myself to, or wished I was 'a bit more like,' become super transparent and I can see their truth, the things they fear, and what's really going on behind the

Insta feed. Emails I receive from people asking me to do something, accompanied by a list of 'all the good things that are in it for me,' almost word-scramble in front of my eyes to show me what's in it for *them*.

AND... I see ALL the opportunities, the pathways, the medicine, the magic, the moves that need to be made. Ideas come through with entire maps provided, and I simply need to execute them. I see ALL the beauty, and it usually comes in the shape of simplicity. Of someone just being really bloody honest. No spiritual jargon, no word salads, no hiding behind a mask, just straight-up honesty about what's going on, what they're thinking, and what they're feeling.

SHE RIFF – LET YOUR INNER TUITION BE YOUR GUIDE

What was once unseen is now seen and cannot be unseen – no matter how much you might want to pretend otherwise – because once seen it cannot be ignored.

You see it ALL.

All the ways you lie to yourself.

All the ways in which others lie to you.

All the ways you've been taught to believe that anything outside is of value and everything inside is worthless.

All the games, the smoke and mirrors, the trickery.

You see it all.

And because you see it all, there's clarity.

SO. MUCH. CLARITY.

You can see where the beauty is.

Where the truth is being told.

Where the gold can be found.

Where the 'real' is available to be experienced.

Where life can be lived and danced and moved and loved.

Where you let yourself be in complete
recognition of your vision.

The vision that's without bullshit
and societal hypnosis.

The vision that's open to synchronicities, serendipitous
situations, messages, signs, and symbols.

Trust yourself, trust your heart, trust your vision.

Your vision is your inner intuition.

Your inner intuition is your guide.

Connect with your inner sight

When your third eye, heart, and pelvic bowl are connected and aligned, you're ALL-SEEING. Previous people-pleasing and don't-rock-the-boat vibes are replaced with 'I see you' vibes – which means you now see ALL the ways in which people may have previously taken advantage of you and your kindness AND you see where people and situations WANT to support both you and your visions.

You can now be open to receive and magnetize ALL the synchronicities, magic, and flow that you deserve. You're a bridge between paradigms – you see what's been, what's unfolding right now, and what's to come. You're an ancestress, a seer of the ancient-future.

All-seeing can also be helluva magical and trippy and span lifetimes, timelines, and paradigms. Just giving you a heads-up!

INVITATION
THE ALL-SEEING THIRD EYE/HEART/CLITORIS RUB

Actual fact: our inner sight and knowing can be activated through touch, pleasure, and orgasm. It's one of the ancient feminine temple arts, and I'm ALL ABOUT IT.

Now, this isn't about me telling you HOW to bring yourself to orgasm. An orgasm isn't the 'goal' AND you definitely don't have to do this in order to connect to your inner sight. But if you are comfy with self-exploration, I'm a major advocate of self-touch and self-pleasure as an opportunity to come in, come down, deeper into your body, your truth, and your power. (With the added bonus of boosting and magnetizing your seer powers too.)

✪   *First, find a comfy space where you won't be disturbed. Have a look around you – know where you are in time and space. Then take a few deep breaths and drop your attention into your body.*

✪   *Give your third eye – the area on your forehead a little higher than the space between your eyebrows – a gentle rub of recognition. Tap your heart gently three times. Next, using a gentle touch, slowly begin to stroke and trace spirals on your face and throat, and then work your way down your body. Take your time. When and if you're called, with love (and maybe lube – your call), bring your attention to your vulva, your clitoris – touch and stroke them in a way that feels juicy and gooood.*

✪   *When you feel connected – remembering that your vulva is a portal for source – when you can f e e e l vital and juicy creative life force moving through your body, close your eyes, bring your attention up your body, through your heart space and to your third eye, and ask: '**What do I need to see?**' Let visions and sensations make themselves known to you. Take your time and allow yourself to BE in the energy of it all.*

✶ *When you're ready, slowly open your eyes, locate yourself in the here and now, and take some deep, into-the-belly breaths. You can create a record of what came through for you by journaling/art/voice notes.*

...

Be forever curious

My mumma told me that my first word was 'why?' I didn't believe her, but I like it as a story to tell. What she actually meant was that, as a kid, I was really bloody annoying, and I'd question EVERYTHING. *Why do I have to eat this? Why is the sky that color?* I've always had a deep need to know ALL. THE. THINGS.

I say this in every book, every workshop, on every retreat: question EVERYTHING. Our curiosity is source power.

In times of distortion, fracture, and uncertainty, although so many of the external structures and systems are outdated and crumbling, we *still* look to them to provide stability and grounding. We can't help ourselves – we've been programmed that way.

However, when we self-source, the invitation of These Times is to come in, come down, into the belly of the pythoness, and re-turn to and re-member YOU as Source-ress. YOU as seer. YOU as medicine keeper. To trust yourself. To open your all-seeing eye and let the energetics and resonance of what you receive from *any* experience, *any* teacher, *any* healer (even this book) be filtered through YOUR body and through YOUR discernment.

If we're not IN our bodies and in remembrance, if our curiosity and discernment aren't online, it's much easier to be manipulated and sold to. Of course, at certain points in our life we *all* need teachers, support, life guidance, and way-showing, and I'm not for one minute saying that we should do ANY of this alone. As I've said, that's how we got into this situation of mistrust and separation from ourselves, each other, and our communities in the first bloody place, and it's *why* I'm sharing Self Source-ery.

This is tender work AND it's what will create rooted, foundational pathways for us to trust ourselves and each other to build relationships and communities, TOGETHER.

So, when you *do* feel the need for outside guidance and support, set clear intentions for what it is you're seeking and then trust your inner tuition and discernment to find the RIGHT teacher and support for YOU. (**FYI:** That will NOT be someone who tells you they've got it all figured out, or that they can fix you.)

Trust yourself,
trust your heart,
trust your vision.

Source Power

*'Her path emphasizes inner preparation,
introspection, and inner transformation...
she carries the sensitivity of sensuality,
in the truest meaning of the word,
finding divinity in the senses.'*

THE GOSPEL OF MARY MAGDALENE, JEAN-YVES LELOUP

When we come in, come down, we can stay IN our bodies for longer and this creates time and space for us to come into a place of communion with the depths of our being.

A place of sensual, fierce, alive, vibrant, and vital agency.

Source power, innate wisdom, your (g)knowing, and YOUR siren song (which has been buried deep within our collective psyche) reside HERE.

From here you can sing the mysteries into being. You can speak the stories of your bones and your ancestors.

Whole and holy

Now, when it's activated, the pythoness, source power, what Hildegard von Bingen (my favorite mystic) called 'viriditas,' or 'greenness' – the divine energy that runs through all living things – is often referred to as 'eros.'

It's a vital, life-giving, creative force which, when awakened within, amplifies your personal DNA, creating *more* delicious, juicy YOU-ness. And if you let it, if you tend to it and nourish it, if you allow your body to become the most fecund container for it, it can, and will, inform *every* expression of your entire life-living experience.

It's a feeling.

It's a pulse.

It's radiance.

It's source power.

Truth-telling, juicy, and vital fluid that calls you IN and DOWN. Into presence (instead of persona) to meet the awakened energetic pulse of Virgin Ma ecstatically birthing herself and new life and possibilities, over and over again.

It's the good stuff. The REALLY good stuff.

It's Mary Magdalene medicine. It's Venus medicine. It's OUR medicine.

It's a guide back to all that's wholy.

Whole AND holy.

A recognition that we comprise ALL the parts – light *and* dark and the delicious spectrum-pulse of mystery that lies in between – brought together without order. Because there's NO order to being a woman who is 'used' (by life, by the Divine, by it ALL). It's chaotic, it's messy, it's real, and it's cyclical.

There's life and there's death. Over and over. And YOU get to be an active participant.

You're alchemical.

A living, serpentine process.

You're full of life force.

You're full. (Of yourself.)

You're the full circle.

Totally holy. Totally whole. All that's wholy.

Let the connection process be s l o o o w. Let it be a delicious and tender unraveling of the stories, the trauma, the conditioning, and the beliefs that don't support your wholy-ness, while at the same time allowing a beauty-full new entanglement to take place between you, Mumma Earth, your felt and sensorial nature, and source power – one that will allow you to become more rooted, more present to yourself and to your wisdom and magic.

Because the more IN.YOUR.BODY you are, the more able you are to amplify the magic of Mumma Earth AND the cosmos, *through* your body. You become a magnetic and radiant force for MORE.

Pleasure as source power

Can you see why we've become disconnected and taught to be fearful of our bodies, our power, and our magic? When I talk about *power*, take a breath and f e e e l into what that word evokes and provokes in your body.

I always joke that I was brought up to believe that a 'powerful' woman was 1980s icon Joan Collins wearing blue eyeliner and shoulder pads, and while I'll ALWAYS have BIG love for Joan, that's NOT the power I'm talking about. Nor is it power 'over,' or the kind of power where only a few people 'succeed' to the detriment of entire communities.

Nope, the power I'm talking about is *source power* – regenerative, cyclical, supportive, sensual, felt, and nourishing. It's *erotic*. Now, much like the word eros, the terms erotic and ecstatic have been reduced to referring only to sex and physical acts of pleasure – for which you can thank pornography – but they're about waaay more than that.

As the US feminist Audre Lorde wrote in her essay *Uses of the Erotic: The Erotic as Power*, 'The erotic is a measure between the beginnings of our sense of self and the chaos of our strongest feelings. It is an internal sense of satisfaction to which, once we have experienced it, we know we can aspire. For having experienced the fullness of this depth of feeling and recognizing its power, in honor and self-respect we can require no less of ourselves.'

Reading and speaking those words aloud feels like warm honey in my mouth. SIGH.

I invite you to do the same. To read this quote aloud and to experience the feelings and sensations that these words, this transmission, evoke in *your* body.

Full-spectrum aliveness

We've been taught that to live and experience life ecstatically and erotically is an indulgence, and that it's selfish/frivolous/superfluous to commit to a practice of coming back IN to our bodies.

We've been taught to reach for and rely on stimulants and false energy that frazzles our nervous system simply to 'get through' the day.

We've been taught to feel shame for exploring our sexuality, which is why so many of us are bone-dry, burned out, exhausted, undernourished, and just waiting to catch the crumbs of all that life has to offer.

Yet to be truly IN your body, with your connection to erotic, creative source power, viriditas, switched all the way on, is to f e e e l and experience and be nourished and powered up by ALL of life. Your personal power as the full mother-loving spectrum.

YOU are NOT here, in this time, space, and place, to simply wait and catch the crumbs of life.

I won't lie, it *does* takes mother-loving courage to commit to full-spectrum aliveness. It requires daily practice to…

KNOW that your body is safe and sacred ground.

Be IN and stay in your body, no matter how much you might want to abandon yourself, numb out, desensitize, or 'escape' (knowing there's nothing wrong if you *have* done that, and are still doing so, because for many of us, these are often acts of survival).

Connect to source, creative life force, and be in communion with life *as* source.

Be real. Not performative.

F e e e l it all and express it all – through the lens of *your* discernment. Remember, not everyone gets access to all of you. YOU, on YOUR terms. Always.

Commit to your felt and sensorial nature.

Choose YOU and keep choosing you in a world where you're told that choosing you is selfish, self-indulgent, and narcissistic.

Become, and perpetually *keep* becoming, a woman who is literally FULL of herself.

SHE RIFF – HOW DOES IT F E E E L?

Do you know how it feels to let pleasure be present?

IN.YOUR.BODY.

To throw back your head in ecstatic rapture?

To laugh, scream, squeal, express yourself
with total glee and delight?

I am SHE who uses ALL of my senses to dance,
undulate, and writhe with ALL that brings me
pleasure, and I want to remind you that with every
breath you take, you can choose to let it become
safe to allow joy, pleasure, happiness, amusement,
delectation, and fun be your guiding force.

Touch pleasure.

Feel pleasure.

Smell pleasure.

See pleasure.

Hear pleasure.

Intuit pleasure.

Sensorial pleasure is the deepest,
most feminine nourishment.

Licking runny honey from your fingertips, the feel
of clean bedsheets on your skin, putting your
hands into mud after a rainstorm, the smell of that
rain on the earth after days and weeks without it,
touching yourself in the ways that only you know how,
a two-hour soak in the bath, laughing so hard you
forget why you were laughing in the first place.

Become the sensorialist.

Be a woman who is pleasure-led, in whatever
shape or form that takes for you.

Be the root-deep, radical, and revolutionary change
that These Times need, and most importantly, require.

Blame and shame her

I think that pleasure, and the medicine it holds, is imperative to navigating a fear-based society that wants us to feel shame and blame for being a woman. One of the many stories from which I've had to detangle myself, and still am to a certain extent, is when and where I consciously choose to make pleasure a priority. Y'see, I was of the belief that when I'm living my life fully and ecstatically – juicy, fecund, creative, sensorial, and sourced – at some point, I'll inevitably need to be/will be punished for that.

Yep, it's yet another lifetimes-old story – one of a woman who dares to prioritize her pleasure, to allow herself to be 'full of it' (and by *it* I mean life, viriditas, juice, source power), to trust herself to be in her fullest expression, only for that fullest expression to be experienced as a threat, as 'too much,' as dangerous, and something for which she must be punished.

I've seen it when a woman laughs out loud in public, deep from her belly, daring to express her pleasure at life. People at a table nearby whisper behind their hands: 'Well, *she's* a bit much, isn't she?' *No* – she's not. She's a woman expressing herself, expressing her capacity for pleasure, and it's bloody glorious.

I've seen it when women are shamed for 'being sexy' or for talking about sex in a pleasurable, unapologetic way. That expression is met with judgment and disdain, yet it's that very expression which will ultimately break the societal shackles that so many of us find ourselves bound by when it comes to pleasure.

Our stories about *why* we feel the way we do *will* differ, yet so many of us are afraid that if we dare to lead a really sensorial, pleasure-led life, we'll be punished, judged, and shamed.

She enjoys sex? **SHAME HER.**

She makes money and dares to spend it? **SHAME HER.**

She expresses her anger? **SHAME HER.**

She values herself enough to say no? **SHAME HER.**

She asks for what she wants because she KNOWS what brings her pleasure? **SHAME HER.**

She dares to be ALL OF HERSELF in public? **SHAME HER.**

I've absolutely NO doubt that between us, we could fill an entire book with ALL the ways in which we've experienced blame and shame for expressing ourselves. AND I don't doubt that, at some point, we've all projected blame and shame onto other women too.

Being full of it

Look, I didn't say this detangling and unlearning was easy, did I? This is a witch wound, a sister wound, a woman wound, and shame and blame are just a few of the tools that have been used for thousands of years to keep us 'good.' And we've been taught, really bloody well, how to use them to 'police' each other instead of sourcing and trusting our own 'value' system as truth.

However, I've a really strong feeling that since you've found this book (or it's found you) you have a KNOWING (even if it doesn't yet have words) that a Source-ress has ZERO interest in being a 'good girl.' FYI: Just to be clear, that doesn't make her 'bad' – that's OLD paradigm thinking, and we're no longer participating in THAT game.

> I don't know about you, but I've spent far too much time oscillating between 'good' girl and 'bad' bitch, and what I know now is that I'm the full mother-loving spectrum.

The Source-ress who is DEFINITELY the full mother-loving spectrum KNOWS that *the* most subversive and rebellious thing to do in response to the lifetimes of shame and blame that so many of us continue to carry IN our bodies (especially with regard to joy and pleasure) is to summon up her mother-loving courage, center herself in her belly-of-the-pythoness truth, flick fear the middle finger and become a woman who is bloody **FULL OF IT**.

FULL of joy.

FULL of orgasms.

FULL of laughter.

FULL of creativity.

FULL of passion.

FULL of love.

There's a lot to work with, isn't there? Take a few belly-deep breaths and pause for a moment. There's no blame, shame, or judgment *here*.

JOURNAL PROMPT

Okay, so let's start with the story – the lifetimes of your own stories – that connects the expression of pleasure with fear of punishment.

Are you able to see what's true and what's illusionary for *you*? What's your relationship with the terms 'good' and 'bad'? Have you ever been shamed, blamed, or what you perceive as punished, for being led by pleasure?

Have you shamed and blamed other women for expressing themselves? (This is NOT an invitation to pick up a stick and beat yourself with it – it's simply an opportunity to explore where your ideas of morality might have been shaped by the stories you've been told about how a woman *should* be and how she *should* act.)

What does the idea of being a woman who is 'full of it' f e e e l like in your body?

Before you try to put any words to it, or start to 'think' about it as a 'concept,' just f e e e l.

Is it sticky? Prickly? Life-affirming? Overwhelming?

NOTE: There's a chance that you've already broken free from those shackles and are now living a life that *does* flick a middle finger to fear, where you *do* live life as the full mother-loving spectrum. And if that's the case, I'm high-fiving and chest-bumping you and taking a deep bow of respect and reverence to your mother-loving truth and courage. Thanks for setting the frequency codes and being a beacon of fierce light for us ALL.

Pleasure as an invitation

Pleasure is me/you/us in our full, sensual aliveness and it's vital and necessary medicine for the remembering and rewilding of *all* humans. It's the understanding that long before we had a fully developed brain, our bodies already had a very strong intelligence, and we STILL hold that intelligence today – the innate knowledge of our sensory and extrasensory abilities.

This intelligence stretches WAY beyond our five senses. Back then, we knew how to navigate and move through the world by f e e e l i n g the presence and energetics of the moon, the stars, the tides, and the plants.

When you're present, when you're IN your body, you're able to see *and* feel how it moves in glorious sync with the rhythms of Mumma Earth, and you're then able to access a vast and thriving potential that comes *through* your body and nervous system.

What if pleasure is an invitation for each and every one of us to…

- Follow something that our cognitive brain has *no* idea about?

- Romance our sensorial nature in true Venusian style? Yep, become the sensorialist – SHE who is in dedication and devotion to the beauty and gloriousness found in ALL things *through* the senses.

- De-armor – with breath, tone, movement, and a HUGE amount of compassion – all the places and spaces IN our bodies where we've tried to 'control' our emotions, 'hold' our ground, and 'protect' ourselves?

- Trust that we don't need to be 'programmed' or 'put under a spell' and that our sensory system knows how to show up and respond? (And that the reality of that is VERY different from socialization and conditioning.)

- Heal and open up magical and deeper states of being *through* our sensory system?

- Enter into a deeper intimacy with who we are?

To be full of it.

To gush and overflow with absolute glorious pleasure that we simply have no bloody space left to continue carrying the blame and shame of the women who have gone before. That our pelvic bowls no longer ache or hurt from the trauma they've been holding that's lineages old, and that instead, we metabolize it, alchemize it, so that it doesn't destroy us but actually makes us stronger and forever becoming.

Don't let them fool
you, pleasure is
your birthright.

The Serpent and the Spider Bite

Although source power is ever-present and always available to us, sometimes it requires nature itself to activate its presence and potency.

In 2018, I was bitten by a spider the size of an *actual* house (I have photographic proof). We had to get the bite checked out, and discovered it was that of a mouse spider, which is big, brown, hairy, and fortunately NOT venomous. Although interestingly, the species did migrate to the UK from the Mediterranean, which is where I found myself a week later, on the Spanish island of Mallorca, watching an incredible woman perform a dance in a village square. (Of *course* I did.)

I was mesmerized as I watched her stamp her feet, twirl and swirl and swish her dress, dancing to an incredible piece of music that created a deep stirring of aliveness, grief, and emotion in my being. When she finished, I approached her and told her that her movement had moved me. She said she was glad because *that* was the idea.

I asked her about the dance, assuming it was a traditional Spanish folk dance, and she told me it had originated in her family's home city of Taranto in Puglia, Italy (she was Italian) and was known as the tarantella, the dance of the spider.

I told her I'd been bitten by a spider the week before – because why wouldn't I? 'Aah, she's chosen you,' she said. 'You're now possessed by the tarantella. And the cure? It's music and dance and pleasure.'

In southern Italy it was once believed that the bite of a local wolf spider was venomous and led to a condition called tarantism. After being bitten by the spider, the victim, known as the *tarantata* (almost always a woman), would fall into a trance-like state of shaking, restlessness, and excitability that was referred to as 'mania.'

The only cure was for the local people to join together in a frenzy of dancing and guitar and tambourine playing. The sounds of the instruments combined to create a healing rhythm that led the *tarantata* to move her body in erratic ways and sweat out the spider's venom.

Ma Malta

The spider bite came at a time in my life when I was living (barely) through what felt like a prolonged dark moon phase. There were various life situations and astro alignments at play in my chart that meant life was 'really gnarly.' (TOTAL FUCKING UNDERSTATEMENT). So, I moved to Malta.

Malta is a place where I'd felt the energy of Ma so strong and so deep; a country I'd written about with such love and passion in my previous books as somewhere I visit on a regular basis to be nourished and loved on by the Great Mumma. A place I *thought* I'd go and live so I could really heal the big grief that I'd been conveniently ignoring – the death of my mumma, my dad, and 13 members of my matrilineal line within an 18-month period. (Because honestly, at that point, I didn't know WHO I was grieving for. So, I disconnected, and I did it really bloody well.)

Until… well, until I arrived in Malta.

I thought I'd spend long days in her many temples receiving codes and transmissions as I'd done so many times before. That I'd walk the land, soak up the Vitamin D, write, dream, heal, vision, regenerate – come back to life.

I thought Ma Malta would hold me, let me curl up in her lap while she lovingly stroked my hair. SHE DID NOT.

Instead, what unfolded is what I now lovingly refer to as my very own spiritual shitshow. (Technical term.) They say wherever you go, there you are. Well, they (whoever *they* are) are NOT wrong.

I thought that the warmth of the sun would heal me. But we arrived during a heatwave that the locals were calling 'hotter than hell.' Brilliant. I had no choice but to sit in the heat of the burn of all that I'd previously ignored. Then storms arrived – gnarlier than any the Maltese had seen in a hundred years, apparently: shards of ice fell from the sky, beetles came up through the plumbing, and the relentless rainfall caused flood damage. And I cried, all the tears. SO MANY TEARS.

These are just a few of the heavily edited 'highlights' of our time spent in Malta. Physically, emotionally, and spiritually it was… a LOT, which is why, after a particularly 'intense' week, I suggested we talk to Ma. We revisited the dream and creation chamber at the Hypogeum necropolis (it's said that entering her is entering a 'womb of time'), paid a visit to the mother temple, Hagar Qim, and walked the labyrinths on Comino and at Ta' Pinu, until The Viking and I found ourselves, at sunrise on the winter solstice, in the Ggantija Temple on Gozo, a small island to the northeast of Malta.

It's the temple site I love most on the Maltese islands (I share the full story of my temple love in *Love Your Lady Landscape*), and it's one that has fascinated me, called to me; one that I've brought many women to in ritual and ceremony; one that I'm pretty sure I've spent many past lives tending to.

It's said, by author Francis Xavier Aloisio, that Ggantija was erected to 'conduct cosmic energy to Earth and, specifically, to draw regenerative energy from the surrounding physical landscape toward the center of the temples.' It was known as a site of renewal, with the serpent – the sign of the self-renewing goddess, of healing, rebirth, transformation, and regeneration – as its symbol. (The symbol that's also tattooed on my left arm. Our left side represents the 'sinister' arts, the left-handed path of feminine magic. The pythoness is the oracular voice that resides within. What I'm saying is that SHE, in serpent form, and I have herstory.)

Heeding the serpent's call

So, I called on the temple serpent of this sacred place for her wisdom and with the deepest love and reverence, I asked: 'WTF is THIS about? This whole experience? It's been a total shitshow – look at us both, we're BROKEN. When does the healing bit happen? Please and thank you.'

And I sat, wrapped in my leopard-print blanket, and waited for a response. ANY response. Because I *knew* that she didn't always respond immediately. In fact, she only EVER responds in *her* time and rarely speaks in words that can be written.

But... nothing came. NOTHING. The Viking kept looking at me as if to ask *What's she saying? What have we got to DO?* Because the whole *let's move to Malta – take a few months out, heal, be in nature* situ I'd sold to him based on the last time we'd sat in this temple together was definitely no longer cutting it.

Three hours passed. It was nearing closing time, and the temple attendants were giving us the side eye, as if to say *are those two still bloody here?* when I pulled my blanket tighter around my shoulders and instinctively placed a hand on my heart and a hand on my pelvic bowl and listened, *through* her.

Come in.

Come down.

Come in

Come down.

I breathed in deeply, past my heart, past my belly, down deep into my cauldron, my pelvic bowl. As I released the breath, I 'saw' a curled-up python sitting at the base of my pelvic bowl. It was dormant and from its center point rose Glastonbury Tor, an iconic hill, steeped in mysticism and folklore, that overlooks the town of Glastonbury in southwest England.

What? I have to go back to the UK, to Glastonbury?! Surely not. I'm sitting in an ancient regenerative healing temple in Malta where, back in the day, people would come to be renewed and revitalized – EXACTLY the medicine I'm looking/asking for, the medicine I NEED more than ever right now – and you're suggesting I go to Glastonbury?

Surely there are some words, some fancy hand moves, I can do to activate this magic. In THIS place. (I've seen The OA, so I know how this works.) And if I can't do that, then why have I been here? What's all this *waves arms around and gestures to EVERYTHING* been about?

As if listening in on my conversation-with-self, the python wrapped herself around my vision of Glastonbury Tor, moved up and through my body, met me face to face, eye to eye, and I heard:

YOU are the magic.

YOU are the medicine.

YOU are the spell.

Oh. Well, that's just bloody brilliant, isn't it? What do you mean by that? Have you seen me right now? I'm a big cried-out mess, and I NEED help.

YOU are the Source-ress.

Oh, FFS!

With that, I grabbed my things, grabbed the Viking by the hand, and left the temple. But what I know *now*, which I didn't know *then*, is that this was all part of the Ma quest. And Malta – the land, her temples, and her elements – was/is the fiercest of Ma love frequencies. Initiatory with absolutely NO hair stroking.

And the serpent? Well, the serpent, the pythoness, has become a guiding force for my own Self Source-ery. Which is why the Viking and I heeded the serpent's call – the call of my own pythoness – and moved to Glastonbury (the mythical isle of Avalon), where we returned to the heart chakra of the Earth, battered, bruised, bewildered, and broken.

The really gnarly bit

I tried to put Lisa back together again, but NOTHING would work.

Nothing made sense. NO THING.

I became scared, fearful, unsure of EVERYTHING. I thought I was going mad.

I've no doubt that you too have experienced THIS place. Sure, the details may differ, but the feelings, the deep-down-in-the belly sensation of *this is messy/I'm going to die/this sucks big ones* IS the same, right? A breakup. A breakdown. When you've lost *everything* and you're on your knees. When you're not sure if you're going to make it. When you don't recognize yourself. When you've NO clue as to who the fuck you are.

When everything you thought was real and true has been burned to the ground, and as you rummage in the embers of who you *used* to be, you find a remnant, yet it disintegrates before your eyes, making sure you don't/can't/won't go back.

Come undone

Sitting in those embers, I was desperate to taste and smell the flavor of who I used to be.

The flavor of a woman who was outgoing and funny.

The flavor of a woman who would take risks.

The flavor of a woman who was fiercely creative – in the way she dressed and in the way she furnished her home.

The flavor of a woman who wasn't scared to paint outside the lines or to make mistakes.

The flavor of who I was before my entire family died.

The flavor of who I was before my unborn babies died.

The flavor of my joy, color, and passion, which died when they died.

What had been left was simply a broken shell of who she used to inhabit.

I tried to sew her back together with red thread.

I stuffed the holes with crystals and herbs.

But… no matter how much I tried, I still kept coming undone.

And as the world, in her own state of change and transformation, became more and more noisy and chaotic, in Avalon, the heart chakra of Mumma Earth, I came in, I came down, I let myself enter the darkest of places and fully fell apart.

YOU are the magic.
YOU are the
medicine.
YOU are the spell.

Good Grief

Grief is a funny thing, isn't it? In the Western world, our aversion to death and grief can mostly be witnessed in our total inability to be with our own pain and the pain of others. It's as if we're 'allowed' a designated, very short period in which to 'grieve' and then we somehow need to 'move on' and 'get over it.'

We're told that's what 'they' would have wanted. (I was told that a LOT. Specifically with regard to my mumma. Except I *knew* my mumma, and what she *really* would have wanted was for me to adorn her place of rest with a ridiculous number of flowers and wail graveside for at *least* a year, if not longer. She was drama personified.)

Very few of us have been taught about death and grief in terms of how to support a person who's been bereaved, either – what to say, and how to honor and hold space for the process. Traditionally in my Traveller lineage, we honor both the life *and* death cycle of a human – we celebrate someone's life *and* we honor them in death. Yet our current cultural and societal experience dictates a heavy emphasis on all thing 'youth,' and little, if any, importance is given to death, dying, and the grief of it all.

In the dark

While my dad's death was a surprise, my mumma's death, four weeks later, was not. And the deaths of 13 members of my matrilineal line – the entire family – in the 18 months that followed meant I had NO capacity to feel, hold, or even know what to do with the amount of grief I was experiencing.

So, disassociation and isolation were my coping mechanisms and they worked really well. Until… they didn't.

I thought I wanted to disappear, but what I actually wanted, more than anything, was to be found.

In the dark, I was confronted by how my body was holding on to grief. ALL. OF. THE. GRIEF. SO. MUCH. GRIEF. I was holding it so tightly. My whole body was an impenetrable armored vessel that set about trying to control EVERY. SINGLE. MOVE. My need to control all the things became all-consuming. I distanced myself from other humans because I thought I was some kind of bad luck spell, a curse, and that anyone I loved, laughed with, and had any kind of fun with would die and it would be *my* fault.

I became overtly obsessed with micromanaging the Viking and his movements, so I knew where he was at *all* times. Holding the tension in my body so nothing could escape and/or fall apart was both physically and emotionally exhausting and meant I'd absolutely no capacity left to *live* life. (And even if I'd had the capacity, I wouldn't have dared to, in case it meant *another* bad thing *might* happen.)

A process of change and transformation

The thing about grief is that it's non-linear. It's messy. It dismantles any kind of structure and order about how we think it 'should' be, which is how I knew that SHE, the Great Ma AS grief, had been working with me, and through me, to create space. Space where grief could teach me and initiate me as a mystery, a practice, a feminine path – as a way to self-source. As meditation teacher Tara Brach says in her book *True Refuge: Finding Peace and Freedom in Your Own Awakened Heart*, 'In the groundless openness of sorrow, there is a wholeness of presence and a deep natural wisdom.'

Ultimately, grief is a process of change and transformation. Yes, we experience grief when someone we love dies, but we can also experience it (and we'd actually really benefit from bringing our awareness to it) at any and every portal of change and transition in life: divorce, miscarriage, abortion, moving house, world changes, other people changing.

> **What I now know about grief is that it's often what my friend Ayesha Ophelia (@ayeshaophelia on social media), who's also a great teacher on all things grief, calls the 'little griefs' – the ones that you feel you might be overreacting to – that act as a portal to access the BIG grief.**

There may also be grief when you menstruate (if you've been hoping you're pregnant and have discovered you're not); there may be grief when you stop menstruating and enter menopause; there may be grief when you experience success and have to let go of old ways of being. The grief experience is unique to each of us.

Becoming forever changed

Look, let's be clear, grief *is* frightening and we don't have to pretend otherwise. It's OK to be fear-filled about the idea of descent because grief, loss, and change *all* have the ability to make us feel powerless and out of control.

The landscape around us is ever-changing, but since 2020 *everything* has changed, and we've not been taught/no one is showing us (in an embodied and true way, at least) how to navigate the unknown, how to adjust our expectations of ourselves and each other. And as a result, so many of us are harming ourselves by trying to be 'normal,' to keep going, and to desperately keep making things work in the same way they did before.

But it's not the same. WE are not the same. If we keep trying to fix something and/or try to make/manipulate/control it to be/stay the way it was before, it's impossible for the rebirth to happen. Rebirth can only occur in the annihilation of it all – when something has fundamentally changed from what it was before.

It's a courageous Ma art/practice to surrender to it. To be willing to receive the potency of transformational magic, medicine, and Self Source-ery that's found in the cycle of death and rebirth. It's also much easier to talk about it when you're not IN it.

I've made grief a practice (see below). I *know*, SO Scorpio, right? I've done this because if we KNOW this place, if we create a container in which we tend to, alchemize, and embody our own grief, in our own being, if we make space for it, if we allow our capacity to meet it to expand, we also make space for the possibility that more creativity, more power, and more wisdom will emerge.

INVITATION
BE MOVED BY GRIEF

This is a three-step practice, and you can do one or two steps or all three. You can ritualize and/or create your own rhythm for it, too. I tend to make time for it on days 28/29 of my menstrual cycle – the days before I bleed – or during the dark of the moon. I do it early in the evening when I know I won't be interrupted. Afterward, I get into bed with a cup of tea and either have an early night or watch something nourishing and heart-affirming on TV to support the integration.

What you'll need

Your journal and a pen; a candle (optional).

What to do

★ *First, acknowledge all the little griefs that you experience – the ones we often don't make space for or write off as unimportant.*

For example, maybe you're a mumma who feels utterly alone in the process. Maybe you feel powerless about what's currently unfolding in the world. Or you get the sense that your opinions are so different from those of your peers that you no longer belong/fit in. Perhaps you'd planned for your life to be a certain way and it's evidently not going to reveal itself like that.

In your journal, write down all these little griefs: draw them out and let them be felt, acknowledged, and honored.

★ *Next, make a playlist that PULLS at your insides. Include songs that you KNOW are so heart-achingly beautiful that you'll want to weep, and/or songs that have an emotional memory attachment. For example, I can't play* Empty Chairs and Empty Tables *from* Les Misérables *without thinking of my mumma. (And inevitably crying because it was her favorite song.)*

Listen to your playlist and let your heart crack all the way open.

★ *Then, find somewhere warm and cozy and gently rub, touch, and hold your belly, your pelvic bowl, your chest, and the front of your neck and throat. Basically, the invitation is to gently and with love, touch the front of your body – the soft body, the parts which, when exposed, are often where we're at our most vulnerable. The parts of us that are so often NOT touched when we go for a massage (unless you're specifically going for a massage that tends to this, obvz).*

Be slow, kind, and gentle with yourself because the soft front body is also where our different life situations and circumstances lead us to create strong, protective armor against the world. And it's often behind that armor, underneath the skin, deep in the fascia, where grief resides.

When you feel that you've naturally come to a place and space of completion, really tend to and mother yourself – make yourself a cup of herbal tea, wrap yourself in a blanket, and allow yourself to integrate and digest all that's come up and moved through you.

So, I invite you to acknowledge the mini griefs, make a playlist, and softly and with all the love you can muster, touch your belly, breasts, chest, neck, throat – maybe touch under your arms and down the side of your body too – and then allow grief to move you. Let it move you AND let it move through you.

Maybe you'll dance, maybe you'll gently rock, maybe you'll cry. I do this practice in the bedroom because sometimes I need to punch and/or scream into a pillow. Try NOT to stop what wants to move through you. But also take fierce responsibility for your well-being in the process.

You may be afraid that once you start, you'll never stop, but this is RARELY the case. If, however, you think it'll help, you can set a timer, or as I do, you can light a candle to mark the start of the practice and blow it out when it's complete.

...

Let grief reveal you.

The Let Go

The real power of grief is in letting it fully disintegrate and dissolve us.

As I experienced my own descent, finding myself in my own underworld, I wanted so much to shout, 'That's enough now, let me out,' and I think, on occasion, I did.

I tried to cut deals with Her. I wanted to force myself out of that process. SO BADLY.

Until… I reached a point where I was just so bloody exhausted. I'd literally scratched my inflamed skin raw; I no longer recognized my reflection in the mirror; and I could no longer maintain the white-knuckle grip I had on ALL. OF. THE. THINGS.

I LET GO. I let all my pieces fall to the ground and I came undone.

I died to everything I thought I knew to be true about me (and the world) and sat in the dark. In the complete not knowing of *if not this, then what?*

I didn't look away. *I wanted to.*

I really stayed with it. *I really didn't want to.*

Staying with it

So often, we want to rush out of the underworld, the darkness, the discomfort. And yet – and this has become my mantra for ALL things – staying with it really is 'part of the process.' When we truly surrender IN to the well of grief (remembering that wherever there's a well, there's source power), there's an opportunity to dissolve and transform. It's where the unbearable can become bearable. It's alchemical.

Don't push, don't force, just allow yourself to be in the deep darkness. It's a nourishing process – being in the vulnerable depths of it all. When we don't accept where we are 'in the process,' we'll often do whatever we can to escape the deeply uncomfortable feelings of being with ourselves.

> **We've been conditioned out of feeling 'depressed' (or feeling *anything*) when it gets 'too much,' and we're often told to 'snap out of it.' Yet staying IN the dark means our roots get stronger, and strong foundations are formed that allow us to grow.**

In fact, and this is WAY easier to say and experience as truth when you're NOT in the darkness and the depths of grief, it's actually really bloody magical. All new life requires death. It's the nature of what is.

But for me, and most probably for you too, that didn't change the fact that it was... really gnarly. In the place where I thought clarity would come and healing would happen, it seemed that all the things I'd ever messed up in this lifetime became BIG and REAL and made me vomit. All the people I'd 'wronged,' all the things I'd said that had hurt others, all the actions I'd taken which, for whatever reason, wouldn't be seen as 'right' came to the surface.

NOTE: I share this because, if something similar comes up for you, or it does in the future, I don't want you to think that guides/teachers/way-showers are somehow immune to experiencing the gnarly and shitty stuff. OR that they're SO advanced, they don't need to 'clear,' 'purify,' and 'let go' – that's NOT true. My biggest wish for those awake to their lived experience, and for those who choose (or are chosen) to speak and share about it as guides/teachers/way-showers, is that they do it 'without the gloss.'

For the most part, I find it *all* really bloody painful. Because being awake and alive to it ALL, taking responsibility for your actions, recognizing what's yours to burn through and what lessons need to be learned, practicing compassion for yourself and each other (instead of making judgments), recognizing what's being projected on you and why, practicing discernment to find what's actually true, AND letting as much joy, pleasure, and happiness in while we figure out why the fuck we're here… well, that is WORK.

No one tells us that. Because unfortunately, the 'wellness' and 'self-help' industry wants to sell us cures and 'fix-alls.' The 'process'? All of THIS? Well, that's NOT sexy, not easy to package, and it doesn't really sell. Yet we're forever in the process of becoming, and more than ANYTHING, we ALL need support with navigating the ever-unfolding, ever-becoming. And we need those who we look to for that support to be truthful about ALL its parts.

Ma's fierce, all-consuming love

I felt worthless. I felt that *nothing* made sense. (It didn't. It really didn't.) I felt there was nothing that anyone could say to me, or about me, with regard to the awful person I deemed myself to be.

My thoughts? They were dark. SO dark. I didn't dare write them all down because I was afraid that I might bring them to fruition. I couldn't, and didn't want to, eat. I'd go from being constipated to what the Viking calls 'sacred shitting.' (See? No one talks about THAT kind of cleansing and purifying, do they?)

It was all I could do to stay with it. To really feel those feels so I might at some point, in some way, transmute them. I sat in the dark with it and I scared myself with how dark my feelings were. I'm proud, really proud, that no matter how gnarly it got, I dared to mud wrestle with the fierce love of Kali Ma. *Again*.

This is NOT the 'let's fix the booboo on your knee and kiss it better' kinda Ma love. No, this is Ma love that will meet you in your darkest places – the places that you may have been told/think/believe make you absolutely unlovable – and she will mud wrestle you into submission with love.

Her love.

Fierce love.

Don't get it twisted – she WILL tell you what she thinks, she WILL hold you accountable, AND she WILL love you regardless.

She'll meet you exactly where you are – whether that's feeling abandoned, not worthy, not heard, not enough – AND she will love you. Fiercely.

Her fierce love is fire. It burns ferociously and from necessity.

It's a protector and it's protective, especially when you're in the dark and stripped back to your bones.

It's here where we're at our most raw and vulnerable, AND it's here where it's most possible to 'come to our senses.'

To activate our inner sight and 'see' what's being revealed.

Our senses are heightened. We have access to deeper wisdom (remembering that it's super easy – easier than it's EVER been – to access information. But wisdom? That's deep knowing that's only ever truly accessed through connection to source, sustained awareness, and fully lived experience). And it's here that we get to really feel what it means to trust our instincts and begin to 'see' in the dark.

The void of NO thing

Look, when your grip on how things 'should' be is TIGHT, or when your inner good girl is trying to please and appease, or when you're trying desperately to control a situation and outcome and your body's tense from holding it ALL TOGETHER, and there's a fear that if you surrender to it, shit will get messy, the emotions might overflow, you'll not be who people think you are or want you to be... the invitation is NOT to reach outside of yourself, try to add a thing, fix a situation, or react.

Instead, take a deep breath, close your eyes, and BE in the darkness of the unknown.

The void, the place of NO thing and TOTAL possibility.

Let it remind you/us that the unknown is KNOWN to us.

It's the fertile ground for creative possibility.

We do KNOW what to do here.

Whenever the moon goes void-of-course, we're in unknown territory until it moves into its next astrological sign.

When day turns to night. When being awake turns to deep sleep. When the season moves into winter.

When the moon goes dark, just as it does EVERY cycle before it becomes new, it's no longer visible in the sky, and we're without its light, plunged into darkness and forced to be in the dark, in the unknown.

We're NOT afraid of the dark, remember? It's where we grow our strongest roots. It's where, if we let ourselves, we're able to rest, repair, and regenerate. To tune out all the external information and noise and instead, turn inward and tune in to our own magic and wisdom to receive our deepest visions and insight.

INVITATION
IN the NO THING

Soften any tense parts of your body.

Close your eyes and turn your attention inward. Don't reach outside of yourself, don't distract yourself.

Feel your feet on Mumma Earth, place a hand on your heart and a hand on your pelvic bowl and f e e e l into the void of NO thing.

Realize and recognize that in this moment there's nothing to fix, nothing to heal.

Can you be with the grief that currently lives inside you?

Can you allow your sensory system to f e e e l what you 'see,' without trying to make sense of it?

Can you simply allow your feelings and sensations to be present?

You can do this because you know EXACTLY what's possible here.

ANY THING.

It's that simple and it's that complex.

• • •

The truth of the matter

Let's be honest, I don't think anyone actively wants to go: *Hey there, sign me up for that exploration of grief in the darkness.* And yet, it's in the darkness of the moon, in the menstruating phase of a menstrual cycle, in the depths of winter, in the dark of the night, in the belly of your being, in the black hole of the cosmos, in our own experience of death and grief that we're given the opportunity to learn and fully experience the stripped-to-the bones bare truth of the matter. Exactly what it is that DOES matter.

✩ Source-ery Support ✩
The Protector-ess

This essential oil blend is nurturing, calming, and purifying, as you dare to show and share your bare-assed self in the world. I created it when I was experiencing the dark (it's good to use for those dark moon feels too) and wanted to scratch my skin to the bone.

Combine pink lotus oil (that shit is expensive, but you WILL thank me), rose oil, and hyssop oil. Try not to smell the hyssop separately because it's very... *pungent.* And use it, and the other oils, sparingly; also, DON'T use hyssop if you're pregnant. It IS super sacred, though, and so good for purification.

You can add this oil combo to a salt scrub with a little nut oil as a carrier and use it in the bath. It also works great in a diffuser too.

...

Ma of the Dark Matter

If you're feeling pulled apart, broken, disconnected, discombobulated, fully IN the not knowing of the in-between, meet Ma of the Dark

Matter. (If you're not, give yourself a big hug for all the times you HAVE been in that place and have survived. Then mark this page for the times when you might find yourself here again.)

Ma of the Dark Matter is the initiate of transformation, and in Her presence, all there EVER is to do is surrender.

Things are often darkest before the dawn and there WILL be a sense of discomfort. If you s l o o o w down, you'll find that there's GOLD in the discomfort – you may not discover it right away, but in the surrender, you allow yourself to be open to discovering it.

Step naked into the ring of fire – drop all the masks, pretense, versions, outdated thoughts and beliefs, ideas of who you are, what you think 'should' be happening in the world, all your judgments about how you and other people *should* be doing things and how you/they *should* be showing up, all the ranty comments on social media, all the instructions for what you *should* say, be, or do in order to be a 'good' person – and surrender.

Surrender it all.

As always, I want to be really clear that everything I share is an invitation. If you're experiencing the darkest of dark spaces, it might be all you can do to get yourself out of bed – if that's the case, take a look in the mirror, give yourself a wink and a nod of loving recognition for doing *that*, and then soothe yourself in a way that feels good for you.

I've said it before, but These Times? The times in which we find ourselves *right now*, collectively, are prep work for What Comes Next. They're a siren call for you, as Source-ress, to receive and gather information (on your terms and in your own way), f e e e l it in your body, and practice discernment in concordance with your deep remembering – the knowing that's outside words and information.

You'll trust yourself to make your own choices, and fueled by your connectivity to source power, you'll act accordingly.

Remember, I'm not your teacher. I'm a way-shower, a guide – someone who shares her own experience, offerings, and medicine as potentiality and possibility to support YOUR process. And I take that role very seriously. But it's YOU, connected to source, trusting your instincts and felt knowing, who gets to reveal YOUR real and cocreate YOUR lived experience.

∼ RITUAL: MA AND THE RING OF FIRE ∼

Are you singing the song 'Ring of Fire?' I TOTALLY am. Go hit it up on your listening device… OK, now that's out of the way, let's begin.

WHAT YOU'LL NEED

A candle (optional); rose petals (optional); your journal and a pen.

WHAT TO DO

First, create a circle of power around you, using either a pointed finger or rose petals, and call in your support team: those who protect you.

✶ Depending on where you are and what's available to you, either make a fire, light your candle, or imagine a fire in front of you. Stare into the flames – real or imagined – and ask for your mind to be clear, your inner sight to be focused, and love to be prioritized. Imagine that around you is a ring of fire. It's cleansing, purifying, a circle of recapitulation.

✶ Either sit with your spine straight or stand tall, and feel a heaviness in your cauldron, your pelvic bowl. Let your belly be soft and your heart be open. If there's any stickiness or stuck-ness in your body, give yourself a gentle shake and then soften.

✶   Place one hand on your heart and the other on your pelvic bowl, connect with your breath and declare out loud: **'I surrender. I'm not afraid.'** Notice any sensations or feelings in your body as you do this. Keep breathing.

✶   Stay IN your body and listen for your own needs. Now ask yourself the following question: **'What needs to burn?'**

Give yourself time. Breathe. Be present. It might get a little uncomfy but try to stay with it. As you feel and sense what the question evokes in your body and where, remember that what you receive may not unfold/make itself known in a linear way.

So, if symbols, colors, or smells make themselves known, acknowledge them and note your responses in your journal; if you prefer to, you can say them out loud into voice notes on your phone, or turn them into art, or move your body and express them.

✶   When you're ready, come back into connection with your breath, your pelvic bowl, and your heart. Then declare the following words out loud:

'I'm courageous. I have mother-loving courage. My heart is big, and I'm here to support the creation of new possibilities that are for the good of all humanity.'

Breathe deeply into your center, your medicine bowl, hold the breath in that space, let it alchemize, feel the heat of the fire, and on the exhale, let the breath be noisy and deliberate. Do this between five and 109 times. Your call.

✶   While you're in this circle of power and protection, if there are any intentions you want to set in motion, to be ignited by the fire, know that this power portal is THE one in which to do so. Keeping your energy high, declare your intentions out loud or write them down.

Then inhale and on the exhale repeat the word 'Ma' over and over until you reach the end of the breath. Do this between five and 109 times. (If you do NOTHING else, do THIS – the Ma frequency is EVERYTHING.)

✯ When you're ready, and your ritual feels complete, give thanks to your support team, blow out the candle, and declare your circle closed.

...

After the ritual, drink lots of water, bathe, eat chocolate, have sex, put your hands in the earth, nourish yourself with beautiful food, do something that feels good. And if, like me, you're a super-sensitive type who experiences ear ringing and dizziness when the energy's high, keep coming down to your center, your medicine bowl, and doing whatever you need to do to stay in your body. OK?

YOU matter

How does the idea/concept of Ma, Mumma of the Dark Matter – this fierce, all-consuming love – show up for YOU?

Maybe you've been complacent, or you haven't felt able/safe to show your true and real expression, and she brings the fire, hands you the match, even, to ignite what's required in you to create and stand your sacred and fecund ground.

Or...

Maybe she meets you IN the fire, where you're consumed by rage and fury, and she holds you there, without judgment, in recognition of all that you are.

Or...

Maybe she meets you in the ashes of all that was, in the afterglow, and reminds you what it was all for: that in the dark of matter, YOU matter.

For me, she shows up as all three, and has been ever-present in the AM (After Malta), where I've had to keep surrendering over and over to all that I *thought* I was, to all that I *thought* I was here for. It's here that I continue to meet the pythoness, a reminder of the left-handed feminine magic and wisdom that's alchemized in this portal.

A knowing that the act/art of death and grieving is a mystical and immense experience that occurs IN.OUR.BODY. Yes, for ourselves, but also for the collective. And the more I/we can gain mistress-ry of it – the ability to acknowledge and soften to previously displaced feelings, all the things that I/we have previously been protecting ourselves from, and then curate and create space to journey *through* them with the intention of becoming all the way alive – the more possible it is to deepen into the experience of life, and call forward the rebirth with fierce, embodied love.

It wasn't until I met Ma at my most (self-perceived) unlovable – when I thought I was 'bad,' a 'curse,' someone who didn't deserve good things like love, babies, family, pleasure, and fun – that I KNEW what fierce love looked, and more importantly, FELT, like.

It's how I now know I can say, with one hand on my heart, the other on my cauldron, as someone who's forever and always in service to the embodiment of Great Ma love, that there's nothing anyone can bring to me, either in a client session or in life, that I don't have the capacity to have fierce compassion and love for.

Why? Because I've been met there.

All my parts were seen and known. By Ma. By the Ma *in* me. By me.

And I was loved hard and fierce in that place. I was loved into submission. I was rehabilitated back to love *by* love.

And I wish that for ALL of us. For ALL humans.

NOTE: I'm blessed in that I know this process as initiatory, but there was a time when I thought I was going mad. (It's why so many of us who associate with the archetypal Source-ress often find ourselves working/seeking/studying that which is unspoken and 'taboo' – we *know* there's something deeper to be discovered there. Or perhaps we hear and experience things, spiritual phenomena/voices, that take us on an impassioned quest for meaning.)

During my many years spent working with women in a psychospiritual capacity, it's become so obvious to me that a lot of women who experience this place, or varying versions of it, either self-medicate their experience in order to 'get on' with life or are given pharmaceutical medication to sedate those feelings in case they 'spill over.'

I'm not against/judging medication, by the way. Far from it. I'm just really aware that women are often called 'mad' and 'hysterical' and then pathologized and medicated when they may actually be experiencing something deeply spiritual and initiatory. And yet we simply have no systems in place to first, recognize the stresses of a spiritual emergence/emergency without confusing it with mental illness, and then, to create sacred containers to hold space for it in the fierce reverence that it requires AND deserves.

It's in the darkness
that we grow our
strongest roots.

Here Lie Dragons

I'll be honest, I've been studying the mythos of the Goddess, tracking the moon phases, my menstrual cycles, and the astrological cycles of the cosmos for a LOT of years, so while I KNOW that the process of 'death' – whether it's actual or metaphorical death, or both – is necessary for the rebirth, you don't quite realize how death-y it gets down there in the darkness until you're really IN IT.

I'd been stripped bare. My body had taken on a different shape. Friends were lost (because not everyone knows how to be IN the darkness and/or how to be with those who are. And you're also not always that fun to be around. So, those who do stick around? They're your people. Hold them close).

We don't need saving

Ma of the Dark Matter, the dragon mother, reminds us that we NEVER needed to be saved from the dragons. Oh no, that's yet another distorted spin on a much more ancient tale. In OUR living mythos, it's here, in the darkness, when we come in, come down, that Ma reminds us that it's time to return to BEING the dragon – primordial, creative, perpetually birthing source power.

Except when you're IN the darkness – and remember, the initiatory experience that brings each of us IN will be different, so please

NO comparing whether your darkness is MORE or LESS dark than someone else's: that's NOT how it works – it WILL feel like it may never bloody end. But it does. It *really* does.

I can say this now because I'm on the other side of *that* particular underworld experience – because let's be clear, it wasn't my first, and it won't be my last – this is the nature of someone who's in tune with the cyclical nature of ALL things. So, ideally, I'd love Kali Ma to provide an ETD (Estimated Time of Darkness) upon arrival, but rudely, that's NOT her style.

However, staying present IN the dark, f e e e l i n g and sensing and 'seeing' our way through it, allowing our roots to get established in the fertile void of NO thing and the uncertainty of it all IS how we learn to navigate the space. And THAT is what's being required of us all as we navigate this current time on Earth – to trust ourselves as dragon mother, connected at the root to primordial, creative, perpetually birthing source power so that we have the strength and resources to rebirth and mother ourselves FROM and OUT of the darkness.

Don't build your forever home in the dark

Now, the dark is NOT where you build your forever home. Sounds pretty self-explanatory, I know, but when you're there, if you stay a while, your eyes start to adjust to the darkness of the dark and it can become strangely familiar, seductive even, to stay a little longer. And then a little longer still.

You isolate yourself, believing that those ashes of who you used to be are where you need to stay, and that there's no way someone like YOU – insert here all the names and labels of shame and blame that you've been dipped and drip-dried in, by yourself and others – deserves to reverse the curse, and well, actually survive.

Yet, an initiation through, and a relationship with, Ma of the Dark Matter is the start of self-intimacy with ALL your parts. To know her is to know that, through your experience of grief, pain, disappointment, anger, death – both real and metaphorical – you've met yourself in the dark. AND you're still here. You're alive. Because you've done this a thousand times before, you've kept score, so that THIS lifetime is the one where you didn't simply survive, but you chose to thrive. The lifetime where you chose to flourish, nourished. (And satiated and FULL OF IT.)

So, don't build your forever home in the dark. Instead, as Source-ress, set the intent, for both descent AND ascent, to become your lived and loved rhythmic experience.

Your magic AND your medicine. Your dance AND your song.

Set your heart as your compass, be IN your body, and be IN ritual and ceremony with ALL of life. ALL OF IT.

SHE RIFF – SET YOUR HEART AS YOUR COMPASS

Shhh, can you hear that?

That's the beat of your heart.

Your unique-to-you rhythm.

It's the drumbeat that will always lead you home
to yourself, to your ancestors, to your roots.

It's the sound of truth, it's the sound
of love, it's the sound of you.

Make your heart your compass.

If life isn't turning out the way you think
it should right now, check in with it.

If you have a big decision to make, check in with it.

If you're afraid, if you're in pain, if the darkness
feels all-consuming, drop into your heart.

The answers to ALL of your questions lie here —
you just have to get still enough to hear them.

Big love and fierce gratitude widen the
expression of your heart and increase your
ability to nourish the goodness that's in and
around you. So, it makes a whole lot of sense
that no matter what's going on in your life
right now, you do more of that, right?

The power of love

Place a hand on your heart space.

Here is where the truth of all existence lies.

You are the keeper of the flaming, ever-expanding, healing heart.

The heart that knows you've been hurt and have experienced pain. So much pain. Pain that means you'll do all the things you can to protect your heart from *ever* feeling that way again. But your heart isn't meant to be shut down — its deeper chambers are each like an ancient Egyptian temple that holds old magic and power and potency that return us to love. Over and over again.

Your heart has the capacity to expand, to transmute, to heal, so tap it gently to remind yourself that you can f e e e l it all and stay present IN your heart.

Breathe IN white light to your heart and breathe OUT a beautiful emerald-green ray.

That beautiful green ray emanates from your body as you breathe.

White light in, green ray out.

You know that…

The power of love will ALWAYS win out. ALWAYS.

So, you stay with it. You whisper prayers of gratitude directly into the face of terror and fear. You're able to feel any darkness weaving insidiously through your system. And *still* you stay in your heart.

White light in, green ray out.

You know that…

The power of love will ALWAYS win out. ALWAYS.

You feel your heart expanding physically and etherically as you use the power of breath and color to take your fears and darkness to the altar of your heart and allow them to be consumed whole by love and gratitude.

The heart isn't to be protected. It's a sacred healing space in which to come into communion with yourself, to feel the pain and terror and experience darkness and heartbreak, in order to expand and grow emotionally and spiritually and come into a place of deep trust that…

The power of love will ALWAYS win out. ALWAYS.

And when you can trust your heart as a compass (I have a compass tattooed on my arm, with true north always pointing toward my heart, just in case I forget), you can slowly, really s l o o o w l y, start to expand to the joy and pleasure of being with yourself, ALL your parts, unapologetically IN your body.

The power of love will ALWAYS win out. ALWAYS.

Back to the spider bite

Had I not created my whole world, I would have certainly died in other people's.
Anaïs Nin

Remember the spider bite? (I told you this book would be a series of woven word threads, didn't I?!) As I said, it happened at a time when I was sat in the embers of who I used to be, wondering: *Who will I become as I rise?* I was aware that who I'd been was no longer replicable. *I* was no longer replicable.

The spider bite and meeting the glorious Italian tarantella dancer who I now know as Marie Rose became a 'moment' in my own Self Source-ery, a 'charming' of my own serpent source power back to life to support my flourishing, rooted-in-the-dark ascent.

When Marie Rose told me the story of the tarantella – the dance of the spider – over a bowl of olives and a plate of cheese, she remarked that, in a world where women are so often told they're crazy, it's much-needed medicine and that we need to remember it. She distinctly asked that I share it in *all* of the ways.

I've since studied the tarantella (I'm learning, very slowly, to dance and play it too), and my question was/is: What if the 'mania' induced by the spider bite was/is our unheard siren call? Our deepest longing unfelt?

What if the spider bite – remembering that the spider is representative of the Creatrix goddess, SHE who's forever creating, birthing, and weaving new ways and worlds into being – was/is my heart shock/ reminder to cocreate a world, self-sourced, in alignment with my own mother-loving true nature?

We change. I, like the serpent, have shed my skin more than a few times. (And that's just in THIS lifetime.) It's OK to shed identities, to be curious, to question EVERYTHING, and to then actively, consciously, with a wide-open heart, come in, come down, into your cauldron, your pelvic bowl, and birth *more* of *your* becoming into being.

∾ RITUAL: WHAT DO I KNOW TO BE TRUE? ∾

This practice/body prayer is for creating a rooted foundation for What Comes Next. For when we've been pulled inside out, when we want to call back shards of power that we've given away – or which were taken from us – and when we may not recognize or even know who we are anymore. Allow yourself an hour to complete this and ask your family or those you live with to be respectful of you and your practice during this time.

WHAT YOU'LL NEED

A candle; rose petals (optional); a comfy cushion; your journal and a pen; a playlist of 3–6 songs that you love.

WHAT TO DO

First, create a circle of power around you, using either a pointed finger or rose petals. Light your candle and call in your spirit team – your guides, ancestors, and those who protect you.

☆ Sit on your cushion and make yourself comfortable. Close your eyes and when you're ready, take five big, deep breaths. Breathe in through the nose for a count of five, hold at the top of the breath for a count of five, release through the mouth for a count of five.

☆ When you're ready, rub or clap your hands before placing one hand over your heart and the other over your pelvic bowl. Allow your breath to remain deep and rhythmic as you settle into your body and bring your attention to the palms of your hands.

Imagine there's white light with crystal-like particles in the palms of your hands and send that light directly into your heart and pelvic bowl. Let that white healing light with crystal particles work its way around your body. Let it fill you up. Let it allow there to be truth and clarity within your being.

When you're ready, anchor that energy firmly into the ground beneath you by placing your palms and the soles of your feet firmly on the ground and stamping or tapping them.

✯ Again, when you're ready, open your eyes, go to your journal, and ask yourself:

'What do I know to be true, in this moment?'
'Who am I right now, in this moment?'

Don't think too hard – your response doesn't have to be coherent. And don't try to think logically, either. Just allow yourself to respond quickly and directly from your medicine bowl.

✯ Come to your feet. If nothing came through in written form, it may do when you move your body. If visions HAVE come through as words, allow the movement to embody this.

Put on your playlist. Start by allowing your feet to make full contact with the ground beneath them. Let the beat and rhythm of your playlist move through your body. Let it move your body in whatever way your body feels called to move and keep moving it.

Gently tap and stroke your body as you move. Be IN your body. If you feel yourself disconnecting, stamp your feet, touch your pelvic bowl, touch your heart, breathe into the space beneath your palms as you move.

✯ When the playlist stops, place a hand on your heart and a hand on your pelvic bowl and be still in the vibration of you and your body.

Now whisper to yourself three times: **'I am loved, I am lovable, I am love.'** In your journal, take note of anything that comes up.

✴   Stay in stillness for as long as you need to. When you're ready, close the circle.

• • •

I invite you to do this practice often, moving your body to the questions *What do I know to be true, in this moment? Who am I right now, in this moment?* – recognizing how different it may feel when you're menstruating or are feeling stressed, or if you do it after sex, or before food, or as the moon moves from new to full, or any other of the millions of scenarios that impact you and your body.

If you tend to be always up in your head and thoughts, it's an act of self-devotion to check in with the truth of your body on a daily basis. Giving ourselves permission to be with whatever THAT is – whether it's feeling scattered, powerless, full of joy, totally powerful, or anything else on the spectrum of feels – helps us to get present to our presence.

We're not trying to fix anything – we're simply recognizing where we're at, acknowledging what we're feeling, being with what is, and remaining connected to our bodies so we can locate ourselves and create; and if and when we call back dislocated power, it has a place and a space to return to.

Back to basics

I don't want it to seem that what I'm sharing here was a Dorothy in *The Wizard of Oz* moment for me, one where I clicked my heels together three times and suddenly, I was able to simply trust my heart as my compass. I wasn't.

For a while there, I trusted NO ONE. I didn't do rituals, I didn't call in my spirit team, I didn't care for moon ceremonies. All the talismans, all the crystals, all the statues, all the books were packed up and shipped out to the charity (thrift) shops and bookstores of Glastonbury; they were positively heaving with my What's Been Before, all of which had shaped the person I no longer knew.

The food I ate, the spiritual practices, the work I was doing/not doing in the world – spiritual/physical/psychological – it was ALL in the ashes of What's Been Before. I was hypervigilant for the longest time, and as anyone who experiences this heightened sense of awareness will testify, it can make the act of breathing and resting – both of which are fundamental for this life-living experience – really bloody tricky.

The Viking, my husband, who's *the* most gentle, loving, and patient human in the world, will tell you that he became an EXPERT in the act of Radical Rest – he even wrote a book about it – by living with me through this particular portal. For a while there it felt as if *he* was my only safe space, and I could only *consider* the act of rest if I was snuggled under his arm.

When we learn to stay vigilant simply to stay alive, we can get hijacked by what therapists call 'trauma brain' – our thinking becomes short term, black and white, and absolute. So, as I sat in the embers of who I used to be, with the soft animal of my body *needing* to know its place and space in the world, it was in the pockets of safety that began under the Viking's arm and slowly got stretchy enough to watch a familiar, low-stakes movie and to drink a herbal tea, that I could begin to breathe a little deeper, begin to sink into rest for a little longer.

It was here that I could begin to locate myself. It was here I could begin to recognize what safety felt like to me as I began a new relationship with who I was becoming. Again, this will look and feel different for each of us, but finding those small moments of rest, a place and space to breathe, sent a signal of safety to my body.

Here's the deal: NOTHING is permanent – when you work with your body, and specifically your nervous system, you *can* rewire your responses. I laid down tracks for new neural pathways that meant I was able to stay IN my body for longer. So that slowly, really s l o o o w l y, I *could* begin to trust my big, beat-y heart as my compass.

The power of love
will always win out.

ALWAYS.

Tending the Terrain

My heart compass led me approximately five meters into the garden. Yep, Lilith was 'exiled' from it, Eve succumbed to the serpent in it, and it was there where I re-membered, revealed, and became my own fruit of self-knowledge.

It was with dirt under my fingernails, tending the terrain of the already established garden of my rented house in Glastonbury (which had once belonged to the man who'd helped create and establish the town's Chalice Well Gardens, site of the magical Chalice Well and Red Spring – totally unintentional, but clearly divinely led) that I began to learn how to tend my *own* terrain.

I've loved herbs as medicine keepers since I was young. My nanna and I would collect them in her apron lap and make teas and healing tinctures from them (I share all about this in *Witch*), but it wasn't until one sunshine-y April morning that I even noticed the beauty-full bright yellow flowers of the forsythia shrub in the garden beginning to bloom.

I went to meet her. I touched her flowers. Smelt her scent. Drank in the vibrancy of her color. I wanted to tend her, love on her, so I started to pull at some of the dead leaves and weeds that were tangling themselves around her.

**With my hands in the earth (of Mother Earth)
it became clear that the weeds and dead
leaves represented my not-met needs.**

At that time and space in my life, I had NO IDEA what I needed or required, and if we don't know what our basic requirements are, how can we begin to meet them? How can you connect to source power if the terrain of your own landscape isn't receptive, fecund, and fertile? How can you be truly nourished (to flourish), if you don't know what it is that you're truly longing for?

Return to what you long for

What I know now is that living in a culture bereft of the Great Ma, grieving my own Ma, and not being a Ma who births babies, meant I'd allowed myself to believe that my terrain wasn't worthy of being tended. That it wasn't a terrain that got to thrive and bloom. And yet, kneeling at the foot of the forsythia, I dared to re-turn to what I longed for.

To meet the mother IN ME.

And when I did THAT, I found Mother in ALL of creation.

✲ Source-ery Support ✲
Make a flower essence

I fell in love with the forsythia and her glorious yellow flowers. I spent a LOT of time hanging with her and looking at her because she's good vibes in plant form. Her presence helped me to feel vital and joy-filled, so I got a nudge from my nanna to make a flower essence from her.

I'll share how I did this – I trust myself and my instincts – but I invite you, if you're called, to make a flower essence with a plant of your choice. Take total responsibility for researching that plant and flower, and to not ingest anything without knowing exactly what it is.

Forsythia's essence motivates the transformation of old, not-needed patterns of behavior – habits, addictions, thoughts. Basically, I made an alchemical elixir for EXACTLY what I needed. Nature really is magic like that.

1. Pour spring or distilled water into a glass bowl.

2. Speak to your chosen plant and ask permission to take some of its flowers. Give thanks and love in whatever way feels good.

3. Gather the flowers without touching them – I use tweezers – and place them in the bowl of water.

4. Allow them to sit in the sunshine/moonshine – either/or both – to infuse.

5. Drain the water from the flowers to create a 'mother' essence. This is the source essence from which you can make 'stock' essences. I make my stock essences in brown glass drop-bottles: I use 1 ml (⅕ tsp) of alcohol (vodka or brandy) as a preservative and then add the infused water to the bottle.

6. Mark the bottle with the astro details and date that you made it.

NOTE: When I make stock essences from the 'mother' essence, I use between 7 and 11 drops of the mother and add it to distilled water. I then take the stock essence daily – seven drops under my tongue. But you can add drops to a glass of water and drink that throughout the day or put drops in the bath if you don't want to ingest the essence.

• • •

Nourish to flourish

Tending the garden gave me the permission to tend to myself. My love of herbs took on one of its many medicinal forms, supporting me, my body, and my lived experience to become a fecund and fertile landscape to fully receive more of myself.

Fecundity is one of my top five all-time favorite words. When you say it out loud, it feels sensual and alive with possibility. To me, fecund ground is sacred ground. It's ground that's been tended, nurtured, and loved on, and because of the intention and attention it receives, it becomes ripe and ready, radiant, and magnetic – for ideas and concepts and anything that wants to take shape and form: a baby, an idea, a business, a relationship, a home. ALL THE POSSIBILITIES.

So many of us perceive, and to some extent believe, that we NEED to be adored and validated, that we NEED to be someone else's idea of perfection, that we NEED instant gratification, that we NEED a thigh gap, and that we REALLY NEED those over-priced fancy yoga pants.

> **What we ACTUALLY need is the root-deep nourishment that's found when we meet our individual underneath-it-all longing and make tending the terrain of what we find there a practice of daily devotion.**

NOTE: If, like me, you've experienced miscarriages, have been told by a doctor that you're 'barren,' have been diagnosed with PCOS, endometriosis, fibroids, or any other of the many dis-eases that women experience, and have been informed by a medical professional that your source of creative power simply 'doesn't work,' I hear you, I feel you, I see you, I witness you.

So many of us feel that we have no voice in response to this, and more of us still BELIEVE that we ARE 'broken' and that we ARE barren. NOT TRUE. Our bodies are bloody magical, and we get to CHOOSE.

We get to choose to devote ourselves to OUR terrain. To listen to her, to read her sensations, her cues and clues – like my reawakened passion for growing herbs – so that we can tend her and give her what she NEEDS. So that we honor ourselves as fertile and fecund ground for magic, creativity, and the birthing of ourselves. OVER and OVER again.

INVITATION
MEET YOUR NEEDS (WITH DEVOTION)

I invite you to consider what you need in order to nourish yourself and become a fecund landscape that's receptive and able to create and flourish.

WHAT YOU'LL NEED

An A4 sheet of paper or your journal, and a pen.

WHAT TO DO

✻ *Take the paper (or use a page in your journal), turn it to landscape, make three columns and head them: LOVE. SAFETY. NOURISHMENT. Then, in each column, list all the ways and things that you'd like to happen for you to feel loved, safe, and nourished.*

✻ *This isn't a quick fix - this is a process. List all the ways that you'd like to create a safe, loved, and nourished environment in which your body can become a vessel, a place of play and possibility where dreams are explored, where beauty is appreciated. So that your body and being is the perfect terrain for idea and dream seeds to take root and form and become.*

You don't have to do anything with this list, but it's important to know WHY you may be feeling blocks, resistance, or fear toward connecting fully with yourself as someone who trusts herself as fecund ground to play, to create, and to manifest.

...

This is how we start to create clear boundaries and allow our creative source power to move through us, with us, as us. And it can only do this if we're meeting and tending to our needs – if we feel nourished and loved. THAT is when we become our OWN fecund and sacred ground.

The chrysalis of your emergence

I repeat, this is *not* a quick fix. Becoming your own fecund and sacred ground is NOT as reductive, straightforward, and without nuance as a meme on social media will have you believe. Rude, I know. Sometimes, in fact *most* times, we need to create space in which *we* can become the safe space.

The garden became *my* chrysalis. A space in which to fortify myself and grow strength. In the same way that I create transitional space and circles for rites-of-passage ceremonies for women, the garden became *my* transitional space. The space in-between.

When I went back to basics, I thought I'd never hold circle and ceremony again, but the garden and my longstanding love of herbs, s l o o o w l y and over time, held me and fortified me and sourced me until I could hold, fortify, and source myself. And when I could do *that*, I was able to trust myself. Trusting myself meant that I could then commit, once again, to taking groups of women through the experience of ritualizing their own transitions and experiences – mumma blessings, baby losses, power reclamations – ceremony creates space for that.

All life long, we experience a series of deaths and rebirths – some small and seemingly inconsequential, some hugely devastating and all-consuming. But each time, with each emergence from one space to another, from one way of being to another, our self-knowing increases as more of our 'real' is revealed and sacred containers – whether they're ceremonial ones or simply the fence perimeters of our garden or window box – are a chrysalis.

A space between safe and not known for nourishment, fortification, ritual, devotion, and ceremony; a space for real integrated and aligned-at-source transformation and emergence to occur. So that, at some point, on your terms and in your own time, you can declare:

'I AM THE MOTHER-LOVING SAFE SPACE.' (And really bloody mean it.)

NOTE: I now have a garden of my own, a physic garden in true Hildegard style, that I tend and sing to – the strawberries LOVE 90s boybands while the tomatoes enjoy my rendition of Salt-n-Pepa's 'Push It' the most. I draw and make art in it, and I overshare about it on social media. It's a reciprocal space. I nourish her, she nourishes me. Together, we plant seeds, grow strong roots, flourish, and bloom.

We yield and celebrate all that's harvested. We make medicine, we heal, we learn. And we also shed. We surrender it all back to Ma. Transitions within transitions. Cycles within cycles. When the process is honored in a sacred container, the emergence becomes less daunting and much more supported.

SHE RIFF – EMERGENCE

Recognize that when you're whole, YOU are the safe space.

Sense that when you're whole, YOU are the safe space.

Feel that when you're whole, YOU are the safe space.

Know that when you're whole, YOU are the safe space.

In that recognition, sensation,
feeling, and knowing, Emerge.

Emerge as a celebration, a fucking fiesta of the
self. Without shame, inhibitions, guilt, and
blame. Emerge embodied. Expressed. Liberated.

Emerge as a woman who is safe in her
body, celebrated, and whole.

> When we become fecund, fortified, and nourished
> sacred ground, we can self-source, metabolize, and
> recognize our own body — not as some out-there
> concept, but as the safe space, the cauldron of plenty
> from which we can emerge, flourish, and bloom.

FYI: When I say *whole*, I don't mean 'figured out' and 'complete.' I mean totally liberated from the cell-deep fear of not being perfect, of not fitting in, of being too much/not enough, and instead being seen and being able to emerge, without the societal masks, as a true expression of all that you are. Your true nature, nurtured. The mess, the pain, the guts... ALL OF IT.

And I don't mean that you can/should emerge right now, either. The planet Venus takes at least seven months to begin and fully ascend after her cyclical visit to the underworld, while the moon takes 14ish days to move from dark to full. What I'm saying is, an emergence takes time, so take *your* time. It's not a 'ready or not here I come' situ. However, if you *are* holding back, check in with yourself. Is this resistance? Or do you genuinely need a li'l bit more time to center yourself, to fortify, to trust yourself, before you crack your chrysalis wide open?

JOURNAL PROMPT

Make a cup of tea - I recommend dandelion, as it's a loyal supporter of the body and will help those who work with it intentionally to take a leap of faith and emerge. You can use the flowers, leaves, or roots - then open your journal and riff on the following questions:

'How can I create the safety of the chrysalis in my body?'

'What feelings show up, and where in my body, when I think about my emergence?'

'What am I leaving behind in the chrysalis when I emerge?'

'What do I want emergence to FEEL like?'

NOTE: When you DO emerge from the chrysalis, when you CHOOSE to leave the garden, YOU become the sacred container. YOU, IN.YOUR.BODY, connected with and living from YOUR center. Your source power.

You are the
mother-loving
safe space.

Meeting Your Edges

When we emerge from the chrysalis, it's inevitable that we'll meet an edge.

Now, I've always been a bit of an outsider – after all, I'm from a Gypsy/Traveller family who exist literally at the edges of society – so edge-walking isn't an unfamiliar concept to me. In fact, my biggest guide in finding the medicine at the edges is Sara-la-Kali.

She, like the Gypsies/Travellers who revere her, represents freedom, hope, self-agency, and sovereignty – values that are often considered 'dangerous' by those who simply want us to conform, to do as we're told and to follow the crowd. She reminds us that the wise women, the witches, healers, and shamanas *always* lived at the edge of the village.

The edge is often REALLY uncomfy, AND there's *always* medicine to be found there. At the place that's not necessarily fully known and understood. Do you know where and what *your* edges are? We often think of them as pain points or the places where discomfort lives, or the parameters of our own center, and this may be so, but it's also where the magic is, was, and always will be.

It's what the witches knew and know.

It's what the Gypsies knew and know.

Fuck, even the Disney character Moana knows it – she desperately wants to know what's at the edge of the horizon.

The biggest edge

Right now in the world, we spend SO MUCH time over-indexing with our eyes on the screens in front of us that we no longer know the potency and magic of what lies in our peripheral vision. The place where we catch the odd fairy spark of inspiration, or flash of future memory. And if you go there, you'll know. If you don't, you never will. Which would you prefer?

> **It's at our edges that source becomes a force. (Of nature.)**

Often, when we emerge from the transformational time spent with Ma of the Dark Matter, as we become MORE of our mother-loving true nature, the biggest edge that we meet is that we no longer fit. (If we ever really did.) It can feel lonely and isolating and as if no one understands you and what you've been through and/or who you're becoming. Be gentle. With yourself and with them. It's a process.

Sara-la-Kali represents ALL of us who feel that we're outsiders, who live life differently to what's considered the norm and/or outside mainstream societal/cultural parameters, and she reminds us that it's FAR more important to be the fullest expression of OUR realness than a version of someone else's conditioned and projected expectations.

It takes rooted and fortified knowing in your values to *stay* present to what is, to *stay* in alignment with your heart, belly, and pelvic bowl, to *stay* connected to source power so that you *can* walk societal edges and your own personal edges while *not* taking the projections of others – which sadly, are inevitable when you're someone who knows yourself, stands your sacred ground, who puts the wisdom, agency, and autonomy of your body before all else – personally.

Our sensorial nature

For a long time, I played down my Traveller roots because I didn't want to be viewed by society in the same way that my ancestors had; so, like my mumma before me, I become a tamer, more-likeable-by-societal-standards version of myself. But honestly? That served no one, least of all me.

So, it was at *this* edge that I began to cultivate a ferocious curiosity AND discernment THROUGH my sensorial nature.

My nanna taught me how to listen to herbs to discover their properties, rather than look them up in a book; she taught me how to smell when food was 'off' (and how to apply that process to people and situations too). Basically, she taught me that our sensorial nature is made up of *way* more than just the five senses we've been told about, and that we are multisensory beings. (She didn't call it that, though, she simply called it magic.)

All our senses have layer upon layer of super-sensory components to them – there's science to back it up, but ultimately, like my nanna, I like to think of these as amplified sensorial magic powers that mean we can see, hear, touch, taste, sense, and experience life at a deeper, often-beyond-words-time-and-space level and frequency.

Fox scent

Now as a Source-ress, I sniff out what I call my own fox scent. (I love foxes and they're totemic to my life experience, ALWAYS showing up for me in times of big change.) Sniffing out *your* own fox scent is NOT the same as knowing what your favorite perfume is – this is the potent sensed 'smell' of who you are, what you stand for, and what you value.

Your fox scent is the 'smell' of what's underneath it all, your mother-loving true nature, and once you've smelt it, it simply cannot be ignored. Nor should it be – it's the smell of your wildness, rooted at the roots of origin.

I've found that my fox scent is at its strongest at the edges of my becoming. When I'm rooted AND there's uncertainty. When I trust myself AND I don't know what's coming next. (Except I do.)

If you could bottle it (which you absolutely cannot) my scent would have base notes of Ma, moss, and mycelium networks; its heart notes would be rose, honey, and self-trust, and the top notes would be source-ery, sass, pomegranates, and potential. It would be called *Eau du Forever Becoming*.

INVITATION
TRACK YOUR FOX SCENT

I don't have a practice or a ritual for developing this – it only becomes available and accessible to you when you honor and recognize yourself as a sourced force. (Of nature.) When you catch a whiff of it, you'll (g)know. It will smell like your deepest longing. It will smell like your frequency vibrating in alignment with the entire cosmos.

It's what goodness and joy f e e l like. It's what nourishment looks like. It's what source-ery IS.

The trick? The dance? The forever invitation when you DO catch a whiff of your fox scent? Track it. Stalk it. Follow its trail. It's a labyrinth walk into YOUR center AND it's where you'll meet your edge. Stay longer in the places that it lingers. In fact, set up a regular place of residence there.

• • •

When we get comfier with being a little uncomfy, when we meet our edges and recognize that it's there where we might just catch a glimpse of our future history, a whiff of our truest fox scent, a taste of our delicious wildness, it's a much more tempting proposition, isn't it?

Now, what if, in that place of delicious wildness, you find joy?

Imagine THAT.

SHE RIFF — CAN YOU LET JOY BE PRESENT HERE?

Joy, often replaced by the more reliable
emotions and feelings of fear, concern,
and incessant worry, is necessary.

Without joy, life isn't being fully lived.

Yes, the world is changing.

Evolving.

Awakening.

But what if, amongst it all, joy is
possible here? Necessary, even?

The places where we feel scared — what if
joy is possible here? Necessary, even?

The places where we feel hopeless — what if
joy is possible here? Necessary, even?

The places where we worry and are full of fear —
what if joy is possible here? Necessary, even?

What if joy is possible here and now?
What if joy is necessary, even?

Can you be open to it?

Can you let joy IN?

Will you recognize its taste and flavor when it's present?

Consider you and your body as a place where joy
can be, where joy can hang out, where you and
joy can dance a bit, maybe even make out.

Joy is a potent power. It's necessary.

Joy is juice. It nourishes us, lubricates us, re-sources
us — it stops us from becoming dry and stiff and
atrophic and unable to be creative and of use.

And right now? What the world needs is for us to
be in our most useful and creative state — juicy,
full up, a heart full of love and resourced.

It's here, from THIS place, that we can think outside
the box, see different perspectives, have compassion,
offer up new and innovative solutions and possibilities.

This is only possible if we let joy in. Not just
once or twice, but daily, ESPECIALLY when times are
hard and challenging and confrontational, because a
full heart and a body that wears laughter and joy
like a familiar, well-loved coat has capacity.

Capacity for growth, perspective, discernment, and
love — essentials for navigating These Times.

Letting joy in

I've spoken extensively about how hard it was/still is to let joy into my life. I thought that if I dared to let joy in, more people that I loved would inevitably die. If I dared to enjoy or celebrate something I was doing, I'd be punished. (I *know*, right?!) The more fear-y I was, the more fear-y I became, making the possibility of joy being present in my body virtually impossible. It was a vicious, no-fun circle. And honestly, living that way? It's EXHAUSTING.

So, if you're feeling the same way, I'm not suggesting that you JUST invite joy in, and it'll all be better. I had to take it SO S L O O O W L Y. In fact, I still am. Feeling, experiencing, and then allowing joy to be a more-than-fleeting experience is an absolute bloody practice for me.

I had to start by imagining that joy came in one of the li'l brown glass bottles that I use to hold the flower and herb tinctures I make, and that I could take a pipette of joy daily. In fact, when I made the flower essence from the gorgeous yellow forsythia in my garden, I called it 'joy' so I could dose myself daily.

Small, titrated moments. So that really s l o o o w l y, it became possible for my body to remember that it's sacred and nourished ground where creative source power flows and where dreams can be dreamed into reality.

Take it s l o o o w

If we stay ONLY in the place of fear or pain or perpetual worry, we stay stuck, we react, we freeze, we lash out. But if we allow joy to come in – if we let joy be present AS WELL – it brings life and vitality and possibility.

And then, if we *can* let joy in, there will be moments, sometimes hours, maybe even days, when we're able to let it consume us. Each and every cell becomes enlivened and resourced and full, and we're able to see the world differently. We're able to allow for a different story to be written about our reality and what's possible.

> Allow yourself to receive. To be a delicious,
> juicy, and fecund vessel of receptivity.
> Orgasm, color in, dance, move your
> body, get sweaty, stay hydrated, laugh,
> go outside, turn off your phone…

NOTE: I know I don't have to say this to you, but I'm going to anyway: experiencing joy and laughter is NOT ignoring or 'bypassing' the fact that 'bad' things happen in the world. This isn't a this OR that situ. It's a this AND that situ. It's recognizing that the world is changing/shifting/evolving AND you're allowed to experience joy. AT THE SAME TIME. It's how we repair and restore the goodness in ALL things.

If you think, *How can I possibly even think about joy when things seem so impossibly bad?* the idea of letting joy in can feel self-indulgent and self-serving.

So, if this is you, and joy feels like a big ask when faced with... everything, I honor you AND I offer this simply as an invitation to explore what joy *could* and *might* be like.

JOURNAL PROMPT

What does joy look and feel like to you? When was the last time you felt the sensation of joy in your body? If you were to invite joy into your body right now, where would it enter? Where would it live in your body? What would it mean to you to be joy-full?

Sometimes, simply entertaining the idea of joy can create a little space for possibility.

Glastonbury Abbey

I remember, in the midst of this particular becoming, catching a really strong whiff of my fox scent while walking through the grounds of Glastonbury Abbey. I'd been planning to spread my favorite red blanket, lie with my belly to the Earth and have a good sob (one of the gazillion reasons I LOVE the town of Glastonbury is that what I've just described wouldn't be an unusual occurrence there), and as I was about to pass the Magdalene chapel, SHE whispered:

'I am underneath your feet. Your power? *Come in. Come down.*'

SHE knew I knew. She also knew I needed reminding. (And STILL need reminding over and over and over again.) Her altar at the abbey is in and down. Underground. Hidden.

I've stood at Her altar so many times. Sometimes alone, sometimes in ritual with amazing groups of women, but that day, as I placed my hands on the altar, I was alone, and I started to sing.

Now, remember that our fox scent can be a smell AND it can be a frequency, a feeling, a vibration – it's representational of what we long and ache for most and you'll (g)know it when you experience it.

I'm really *not* a singer – although after a gin or three, I'm always the first on stage at *any* karaoke opportunity – yet there at Her altar, I sang a song through me that felt timeless and ancient. I mentioned earlier that I didn't speak during a few of my formative years, and I've explained in previous books how I still struggle with speaking out loud, so this act of what felt like devotion – to me, to Her, to us all – felt big.

And it kept happening. Sometimes I'd know the song, sometimes I wouldn't, and what I noticed was that I didn't care how it sounded. I simply trusted how it *felt*.

It felt like an unraveling.

A cracking of ancient codes at a cellular level.

A deep knowing.

Which was/is the medicine for me. For you. For us all.

Come in.

Come down.

And sing YOUR siren song.

Showing up. On YOUR terms. In YOUR time

Look, self-trust is complex. Fact. There's so much unlearning to do AND it's entirely possible to return to our true and real nature by reinhabiting our bodies and remembering the magic that's held there.

I presence everyday life as ceremony. I'm curious and I question what I'm feeling, sensing, and experiencing in and through my body, every day. Why? So that I don't abandon myself, my body, and its belly-and-bones deep wisdom and knowing.

Slowing down and listening to my body meant that I was able to recognize all the places where I'd stuck massive sticky plasters over a really painful gash. Slowly, one by one, I peeled them back, exposing them to the light, and I did what needed to be done to help them heal.

> I let myself get curious about what
> REALLY needed to be healed. Then
> I dared to let it be revealed.

I say *dare* because it's brave to reveal what's behind the pain/hurt/ shame/blame you may experience.

Pandora's box

Some may compare this to the Greek myth of Pandora and her box, thinking that if we get curious, we'll unleash a whole lot MORE pain and misfortune – we're scared of what we might find.

But remember, Pandora's box ACTUALLY held the truth, and the truth is our source power. The dudes who wrote the myth wanted us to believe that Pandora made the world 'bad' because she dared to be curious, but it's time for us to rewrite *that* myth too. It's time for us to recognize that opening our own Pandora's box is *how* we reclaim our power as oracles, medicine keepers, witches, and healers. So, open it up and take it back, I dare you.

Acknowledge the pain, the hurt, the shame, and 'see' with your oracular vision what is asking to be healed; track your fox scent to find what it is you ache and long for. When you allow yourself to feel it – to stay with the pain and no longer run from it – you take back your power, you recalibrate, and you make space for feminine repair and healing at the deepest level.

Show up as YOU are

Any time we stand in our power and light, say no, refuse to conform to societal/patriarchal norms, it will make anyone who *isn't* doing that, uncomfortable. VERY uncomfortable. And this creates projections, distortions, and power plays.

We're living in times where people think it's OK to school others on how to 'show up' – on what to say and how to act. Finger pointing, judging the 'process.' Nuh-uh. That's NOT how it works. HOW you show up and what you show up for is ENTIRELY up to you. When I'm asked for the gazillionth time, 'Who do you think you are?' I say: A WOMAN. SHOWING UP. AS SHE IS. (Might get that put on a tee.)

> No one gets to tell you HOW to show up, and if they try, ignore them, because no one gets to decide on the how – that's different for each and every one of us.

Some may be fierce activists, while others will create words and art; some will birth babies and plant vegetable patches; some will gather in circles to raise consciousness through ritual and prayer, while others will paint nails and listen to the problems of those sat in front of them. And some may manage, for the first time in a week, to get up in the morning and take a shower... You get the idea, right?!

Let your passion – your anger, rage, and grief for the injustices in both your own world (and don't let anyone belittle/judge/try to reframe what that is for you) and THE world – be turned into art, and words, and love and vulnerability, and sharings, and offerings, and medicine.

A return

Self Source-ery is a return.

A return to our knowing.

A return to our intuition.

A return to our wisdom.

A return to what makes us strong. (And not necessarily muscular or need-to-hold-it-all-together strength; no, I'm talking about the strength, fortification, and resilience that comes from knowing and trusting all that we are, and all that we're about – deep down in the belly of the pythoness.)

A return to your magic.

A return to your re-membrance of you and your pelvic bowl, as a cauldron and container, to potentize and cultivate your feminine magic.

A return to knowing source as a magnetic force.

A return to holding your unique-to-you vibration and frequency without fear.

It's a return to nourishing and nurturing yourself for no reason other than to let it f e e e l really bloody good. (Which, no matter how much we're told it's selfish and indulgent, is a magical practice that will create healing ripples through entire timelines and paradigms.)

It's a return to the sacred feminine art of discernment – part of your source-ery is to know, like every good burlesque dancer, when to conceal and when to reveal. YOU get to choose.

You choose the volume of your magic and how much of that you wish to share with the world.

It's a return to knowing that decisions are best made by the people affected by them.

It's a return to how fucking powerful you are.

So, call back your power from all the places it's been leaky, set fierce and loving boundaries – in fact, let's call them what they really are, *standards* – and create and live your life from the deep and real (g)knowing that YOU ARE POWERFUL.

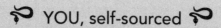

YOU, self-sourced

YOU become intimate with the cycles of death and rebirth.

YOU meet the pythoness – your oracular wisdom, your deepest knowing.

YOU shed, like the serpent, identities, thoughts, beliefs, and stories you've been told and sold, to reveal MORE of who you are.

YOU return to the simplicity of what's real and what's necessary.

YOU trust your body as fecund and sacred ground

YOU live from your center, your power, your truth, on *your* terms.

YOU s l o o o w down and listen to what your body needs and wants (knowing that it's always subject to change).

YOU trust that you, full of it, well nourished, and present to your presence, ripple into EVERY aspect of your life.

YOU realize and recognize that you are your responsibility.

Let your body
be an altar
and live your life as a
devotional ceremony.

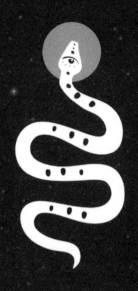

PART III

Remember Your Magic

The mistress-ry of your mysteries, knowing your flow, and living your rhythms.

Mistress-ry of Your Mysteries

Yes, magic CAN look like spells, incantations, bubbling cauldrons, and howling under a full moon – I'm a witch so I have BIG love for that – but Self Source-ery is feminine mistress-ry. It's the magic that you've NOT been taught to believe in: it's the magic of YOU.

The magic of YOU

The magic of YOU connected, at source. (With the knowledge and realization that it can never be taken from you. Not EVER.)

The magic of YOU reclaiming your body, your power, your oracular knowing. (In a system where you've been taught to give your power away.)

The magic of YOU holding both the dark AND the light, power AND love. (It's possible and it's necessary to be a place and space of duality. At the same time.)

The magic of YOU, contradictory, chaotic, paradoxical. Consistently inconsistent. (It's in the chaos of contradiction and paradox that innovation and rebirth can occur.)

The magic of YOU connecting to the land, growing your own plants, herbs, and food. (Because when we tend the earth, we're also tending *our* roots, coming back to ourselves, our bodies, our ancestors, and healing.)

The magic of YOU sourcing your own spring of well-being. (Because when you're full of it – life, vitality, viriditas – the overspill becomes magic and medicine for EVERYONE. Yep, everyone benefits when you're full of it.)

The magic of YOU in tune with, and led by, YOUR rhythm, listening to and singing the expression of YOUR siren call. (Because Self Source-ery is both an art and mistress-ry of your own mysteries – led by your instinctual nature in sync with your rhythmic intelligence – there are times to reveal and times to conceal; there are times to be seen and times where you need to turn your magic all the way down. You KNOW.)

The magic of YOU present to the power of your presence (and letting that be ENOUGH).

The magic of YOU as a living mythos for THESE TIMES (because your aliveness isn't something to 'learn,' it's a labyrinth walk deep into the center of your body, to re-member new and necessary storylines that transcend timelines).

The magic of YOU as a magnetic force, rooted in and aligned with Mumma Earth as power source, to dream, birth, become and radiate a new emergence. A new possibility. (Systems and ways of being are dying and we have the power to repair and regenerate so that we can cocreate new ones. It's *time*.)

You/me/we are the Source-resses and when WE are sourced, the world will be sourced.

☆ Source-ery Support ☆ Mugwort tea

As we move into the terrain of our magic, I invite you to brew a cup of mugwort tea, just as my nanna did. Mugwort is usually the first herb to appear in my garden in spring, and it has MANY medicinal properties. However, I love it mainly because it helps me to remember MY magic and because it's been my main plant ally in the writing and sharing of this book. EVERY time I sat down to write, I drank a cup, because mugwort is a seer's best friend.

As a Venus-ruled herb, mugwort is feminine in nature, and it's useful for supporting us in seeing and visioning our way through the often messy transitions we experience as we move through life. (It's especially brilliant during the transition between menstruation and menopause.) Mugwort is a nerve tonic and a diuretic, and it's considered good for the digestion; it's also a uterine tonic and can be safely taken over long periods of time, *except* during pregnancy.

I dry mugwort leaves and burn them alone as incense – be warned, the smell is pungent – and the herb can be used alongside sage, mullein, and motherwort in a blend to drink as a tea, smoke, or bathe in. Or all three.

I LOVE baths, especially intentional herbal ones, but for the purpose of our current Self Source-ery quest and labyrinth walk together, let's make a cup of mugwort tea. Add two teaspoons of dried mugwort leaves to boiling water and let them steep for 10 minutes. Mugwort solo tastes very bitter; yes, that's part of its medicine, but I always add a spoonful of honey.

Mugwort can support your visions and dreams and when drunk with intention, it can sometimes take you into a deep meditative or trance-like state or activate vivid dream time. I usually make a cup before bed, or before taking a medicinal 'journey' nap.

Before drinking the tea, set a very clear intention, something like: 'I drink this tea to remember my magic.'

...

The assignment is alignment (and refinement)

Yep, I know we've been taught to follow systems, 'listicles,' and five-point plans that tell us what to do, what to buy and how to apply, but when you remember your magic, you know there's NO one-size-fits-all solution and that how it is for you may be totally different to how it is for someone else.

Which is why Self Source-ery is NOT me telling you what to do. It's you, re-membering, descending, down through the layers of your body, connecting with the mysterious force, source – the primal spark of intelligence that informs EVERY living cell – f e e e l i n g into and trusting YOUR oracular body wisdom and sensorial superpowers to let you know what feels real and right and liberating for YOU.

You're a self-sourced, magnetic, pulsing force that syncs with ALL of life – through your rhythmic and cyclical intelligence – to create right alignment.

Your life 'sauce' is
a magnetic force,
direct from source.

Know Thy Cyclical Self

Self Source-ery has been/is/forever will be my commitment to care for myself. I wanted to become fortified – mentally, spiritually, physically, psychologically – so I could fully balance, hold, contain, and potentize my remembered magic. It's meant connecting deeper with my body than I ever have before. I've become a s l o o o w and sensual life live-er so I can really be – and more importantly, stay present to – my presence.

In the past, I was quick to abandon myself. My magic – both conscious and unconscious – felt too big, too much. And I felt too big, too much. Faced with grief, ALL. THE. GRIEF, my nervous system flooded, and I became overwhelmed. My body simply did NOT have the capacity to hold it. I didn't recognize myself, and I didn't recognize others. I didn't know *how* to be here. I thought I was an awful person, so I disassociated.

So, choosing me and showing up for me (as Self Source-ery), regularly and on purpose, has been a true act of care and devotion, one that's allowed me to s l o o o w l y rebuild a relationship of trust with my body. And now that I trust her, I can listen to her. I can f e e e l and sense what lives within, HOW she needs to be nourished and satiated, and without pressure, I source.

My sensorial nature is now awake and online and it helps me to f e e e l the full capacity of alive-ness – joy, gratitude, compassion, love, sorrow, grief. I'm able to celebrate the wins (my own and those of others). I'm able to hold space for the inevitable struggles (my own and those of others).

I dance and sing and cry and I'm present to it all. I continually create and cultivate space in my being for more of my mother-loving true nature to become. (Knowing that I'm *forever* becoming.) It's ancient healing *through* knowing and caring for my body.

Introducing the cyclical SHE-scape

Knowing your body, its shape and form, your tendencies, your patterns is... EVERYTHING. All the information, and more importantly, all the wisdom, about ourselves that we *ever* need to know and access – from our monthly hormonal changes and our responses to music, touch, and lovers, right through to the deep longing to return home to our remembered magic and truest nature – is unraveled and revealed *through* our experience of natural rhythms and cycles.

Yep, our bodies are deeply tuned in to the cycles of nature, the seasons, the sun, the moon, the elements, the cosmos. However, we've been conditioned to ignore our cyclical nature, and instead, we multitask, feeling that we must do it ALL in order to be 'good' and/ or successful. We're told to trust external teachers and voices rather than our own body and its sensorial wisdom, and in the process, we've cultivated a very linear, goal-orientated existence.

One where we've lost our connection to the magic and power that we experience when we have a deep awareness and knowing of who we are through the lens of our cyclical nature.

Inner and outer landscapes

Since my mid-20s, when I was diagnosed with PCOS and endometriosis, I've tracked, mapped, and really *stalked* my creativity, my sexuality, my true nature, my entire lived experience *through* the cyclical lens. Through my body and her sleep patterns, menstrual cycle, and energy levels. Through the cycles of the moon, the planets, and the Earth-based Wheel of the Year and her seasons. We experience numerous natural cycles that weave and unravel throughout our being at any one time, and I call this the cyclical SHE-scape.

It refers to the **outer landscape**, for example:

- The season outside your window.

- The ground on which you're standing – what's it made from? Chalk? Concrete?

- The placement of the planets and the stars at any given moment.

And the **inner landscape**, including:

- Your breath – is it shallow and fast, or deep and long?

- If you experience a menstrual cycle, which phase are you in? Which day are you on?

- Which phase of womanhood are you currently experiencing?

- Where are you at, physically, mentally, spiritually?

Your lived experience as rhythmic intelligence

Rhythms and cycles impact our lived experience, which is why I'm obsessed with tracking, mapping, and journaling the lived experience in *response* to the cyclical SHE-scape.

This practice involves making a daily assessment of our current terrain – surveying the inner and outer landscapes: the rhythms and cycles that are unfolding and spiraling at any given moment. It's also a practical AND beautiful way to get curious about what's *actually* going on in your body: why you do the things you do, and *how* you can work *with* your rhythmic intelligence rather than against it.

Tracking and mapping our lived experience through the lens of our SHE-scape is a potent spiritual and embodying practice because look, that societal spell will continue to try to make us believe that *everything* is a constant stream of production and consumption. But the reality is that we're NOT machines. Your productivity, joy, vitality, and experience of life *isn't* about your willpower and how much you can 'get done' – it's about the resources you have access to in that specific moment, plus the context of the life you're currently living and experiencing.

So, I invite you to see this as both experimentation and exploration. An opportunity to be present with, get curious about, and be fascinated by what's going on for YOU.

NOTE: When talking, sharing, and teaching about our cyclical nature, the rhythmic intelligence of ALL THINGS, and our relationship with the natural world, I've found that we've been SO heavily programmed, we'll even try to find ways to turn *this* into a protocol, a system, a to-do list. (Only to then get really pissed at ourselves when inevitably, for whatever reason, our own experience doesn't align with what we've been told *should* happen in each cycle and phase.)

So, tracking and mapping your SHE-scape should NOT be used as yet another way to measure how 'well' you're doing at life. It's not a disciplined practice because I care VERY little for discipline. I'm FAR more interested in devotion – a devotion to our bodies and our rhythmic intelligence as a way to be present to, and get to know, what's going on for US. Consider it a subject-to-change daily snapshot of your current lived experience, *through* your body.

Cyclical Self Source-ery

Tracking and mapping your SHE-scape – both the inner and outer landscapes – is cyclical Self Source-ery and it gives you access to so many sets of highly practical AND deeply spiritual keys and codes.

As I've found, with each and every cyclical turn, you'll learn more about yourself, about your body, your tastes, your tendencies, and the more you learn, the more you'll be able to fully own and claim WHO you are. You'll be able to take up space, care for yourself without guilt or fear, and live your life in ways that feel totally aligned and meaningful to you.

Unfortunately, the over-culture has deemed natural rhythmic guidance systems like this obsolete, and instead we've been reprogrammed to follow a prescribed calendar – one that operates on seven days a week rather than following the timings of our bodies in accordance with the timings of nature and the planets. But we can reset this.

> We can realign with nature and her rhythms, with the seasons, the elements, the moon, the menstrual cycle, the planets. We can listen to the rhythms and let them become supportive ancient-future 'maps' for our source-ery.

Yep, cyclical wisdom is the foundation of the way I self-source. Working with the ebb and flow of the phases of the cyclical *outer* landscape allows me to be connected to my ever-changing cyclical *inner* landscape: my emotional, physical, and mental terrain. This helps me to recognize what I need to feel resourced, vital, and fully alive in each phase.

How you choose to do this is TOTALLY your call. PLEASE don't let it become another thing to 'do.' My advice? Feel into what I share and notice where you're pulled to most. Your body is a sacred and ceremonial landscape which, when tended and nourished, direct from source, creates presence. Your presence is powerful and emits a true-to-you frequency that's magnetic.

NOTE: One last thing, please, for the love of Joan of Arc and Lizzo, don't let anyone tell you that getting to know yourself, being endlessly fascinated about discovering more about yourself, is wrong. This is yet another move in the patriarchal playbook: make women think that self-interest and self-care are indulgent, selfish, even narcissistic, so that we continue to give, never taking the time to rest, recalibrate, and fully receive; so that we ultimately break down and/or burn out and find ourselves hating our bodies.

So, let's remember how magic we really are through a cyclical lens. Let tracking and mapping the SHE-scape be an act of cyclical source-ery, self-love, and deep devotion. A way for you to remember, reconnect with, reclaim, and revere YOUR power and presence.

Let your magic reveal
itself as you return to,
and fully experience,
the natural rhythms
and cycles of your body,
Mumma Earth and
the cosmos.

Tracking and Mapping Your SHE-scape

There are natural cycles that map and moment-mark the most auspicious times for everything in life. Among these are the cycle of life, the four seasons, the phases of the moon, and if you experience one, the phases of the menstrual cycle, which can be tracked and mapped individually, and most importantly, woven together, to support a life that's in sync with the rhythms of nature to which we're *all* connected.

SHE cycles

Tracking and mapping these natural cycles – which I lovingly refer to as SHE cycles because they bring me into deeper relationship/ devotion with the SHE in me, my source power – offers us the opportunity to draw insights and superpowers from each one and create a container for our own cyclical source-ery.

The life cycle

As we journey through the cycle that is THIS lifetime, we move through distinct archetypal phases. With reference to girls and women, these archetypes are often called Maiden, Mother, and... wait, what's next? Western society is quite simply ageist, and we care very little for women after what's considered midlife, deeming them no longer useful when they aren't 'pretty,' 'sexy,' 'mothers,' and 'producers.' So, we call the next life phase Crone. Yep, that's it, women move from the 'Mother' to the 'old' woman.

I love nothing more than to subvert and disrupt ideas that are restrictive and prescriptive, especially when it comes to how we 'should' live and experience life, BUT I do get that archetypes are a super-useful way to explain models of behavior that can influence, support, and shape the human experience. So, over the years, through my own experience and from working with thousands of women, I've re-imagined those archetypes to *support* our Self Source-ery.

The archetypal and energetic phases of womanhood

We cycle through at *least* four main archetypal and energetic phases of womanhood, and I refer to and witness these expressed as...

- **Minx** – yes, she's young; yes, there may be a naïve innocence, AND it's here, at the transitional point between girl and woman, menarche – first bleed – that she's discovering her magic. She's playful, risky and frisky, fun, cheeky, full of energy, curious and adventurous, exploring her cunning and her wiles as a way to navigate the world.

- **Creatrix** – yes, she *may* be a mother, but she doesn't have to be. When we move into what's often referred to as the 'childbearing years,' we actually have the potential to create ANYTHING – see why this phase needed a Self Source-ery rewrite? It's when we enter the mistress-ry of our magic – we cultivate a deep understanding and connection with source power through our bodies and we hone it, test it, and cocreate a fully lived experience.

- **Charmed *and* Dangerous** – this is a phase that's not often spoken about, and when it is, it's referred to as 'wild' because it *can* be unpredictable. If we experience a menstrual cycle, it's when it may start to change rhythm. If we *do* have children, it's potentially when they start needing us less. It's a transitionary time and if you're not prepared for this particular transition – and Western society definitely does NOT want you to be – you can feel as if you're without a place and space in the world. Yet it's here, in the uncertainty, that the source-ery gets strong. Some call it a midlife crisis, or the Uranus half return, or perimenopause; I call it the time when you care much less about what people think and move from the mundane to the mystic; it's when you're asked to put into practice the mistress-ry of your magic.

- **Wise Crone** – I keep the word crone because, along with terms like 'witch' and 'hag,' we're reclaiming, celebrating, and revering it. We're so quick to write off our old people, yet when we become the Wise Crone we ARE the mystic, the medicine keeper, the (g)knower of magic. If we experience a menstrual cycle, it's when we stop bleeding, because we no longer NEED to – we've gathered all the wisdom from the bleeding years and are in our seat of power, mistress of our magic.

What if *these* were the archetypes that were available to us as we moved through our lives? These phases of womanhood *could* be marked by age, but that would assume there's a set timeframe for when a woman moves from one to the next, and there isn't. It's *all* broad brushstrokes that create the outlines of a map to which YOU get to add details and marker points. I told you that NOTHING about Self Source-ery comes pre-packaged, didn't I?

The four seasons

The Viking and I met through our deep love and respect for the natural world, and our entire approach to life since then has been formed and shaped in collaboration with the Earth's seasons:

- **Spring** – Growth
- **Summer** – Bloom
- **Autumn (fall)** – Harvest
- **Winter** – Recovery

While we both follow different, yet super-aligned, spiritual paths, Mumma Nature and her seasonal transitions are at the core of our lived rhythms and experience. We eat, when possible, in concordance with what produce is available to us in each season; we spend the winter months in our creative caves, and in spring and summer we socialize, share our creative endeavors, and become more available to the outside world.

Anytime I fall apart and come undone, it's Her seasonal rhythms that remind me that there's a time for everything – a time to rest and recover, a time to grow and bloom, and a time to reap all that's been sown. It's a reminder that NOTHING is permanent, that death creates new growth, and that you're not meant to bloom ALL the bloody time.

For everything there's a season, and it supports me to put myself back together again. If ever I forget, I spend time sitting with my back against a wise yew tree in the summer sunshine; when my nervous system is overwhelmed, I lie belly to the forest floor and let Her hold me; I watch the ebb and flow of the ocean as a meditative practice; I tend to my herbs and make teas and tinctures in tune with Her relationship to the sun and the moon and the seasons of the year.

The phases of the moon

Many of us, myself included, are enchanted by the moon and her magic. If you've read any of my previous books, you'll know that I'm OBSESSED with La Luna. She's been a guiding force for me since I was a child, and all the women in my matrilineal line loved on her hard.

My mumma was what's known in the Gypsy/Traveller tradition as a 'sky reader.' She didn't concern herself with the angles and degrees of astrology, but instead, she 'felt' the planets and constellations – she knew their correspondences with the seasons and would literally, like the temple priestesses, read the sky. This is what our ancestors did for millennia, and temples were created for this specific purpose.

Today, we can study astrology and astronomy in all its forms – I have and still do – yet the way my mumma did it? Well, that was a bit less formal, and a LOT more inner tuition and instinct-led. I didn't learn NEARLY as much from her as I'd have loved to while she was alive, but she *did* teach me how to find constellations in the sky, to know what the moon was doing at any given moment, and to witness Venus as both evening and morning star (and to feel the difference of both in my body).

My mumma very much hid and denied her witchy-ness, and I get it – people have highly romanticized views of Gypsies and Travellers, particularly those on social media who appropriate terms like 'exotic' and 'carefree' when the reality for most of us is racism and discrimination. Add magic-making, stargazing, and the gift of 'sight' to the mix and it's NO wonder that my mumma wanted to conceal her magic and try to 'fit' in.

One thing she never hid or denied though, was her connection with the moon. This has led, inadvertently, to the moon becoming one of the most personal, potent, and powerful restorative tools in me, reconnecting with my body and remembering my magic.

The four main lunar phases are:

- **Waxing moon** – What's your potential? Ideas and intentions.

- **Full moon** – What wants to be manifested? Creativity and manifestation.

- **Waning moon** – What needs to change? Editing and analysis.

- **Dark moon** – What needs to be released? Let go and dream.

Of course, you can do moon magic and spells to manifest when La Luna's in her fullness (I deffo do), and of course you can put water and crystals out to be charged by her magic (I deffo do), but the most powerful thing my mumma taught me to do when the moon was big and bright, was to look to her as a prompt for self-reflection.

I've found that in each of her phases – and this is also true of the phases of womanhood, the seasons, and the menstrual cycle – the moon holds cues for us to 'see' and experience ourselves. Basically, if you let her, the moon can be a glorious reflective mirror of your wants and needs as you experience each phase. Consider it lunar therapy – my favorite kind.

The phases of the menstrual cycle

It's NO secret that those of us who have a womb and menstruate, or who have experienced a menstrual cycle in this lifetime, have at some point probably cursed our period, found it annoying, been shamed for it, been embarrassed by it, and/or generally found it really bloody inconvenient. Pun TOTALLY intended.

Yet we experience between roughly 350 and 500 menstrual cycles in our lifetime – the number depends on various factors that can include pregnancy and health issues – and every one of them has the potential, through each of its four distinct phases, for us to listen to our bodies and become better acquainted with ourselves.

The phases of the menstrual cycle are:

- **Pre-ovulation** – estrogen rises, an egg is prepared to be released

- **Ovulation** – estrogen peaks, an egg is released

- **Pre-menstruation** – progesterone is produced, peaks, and drops in preparation for potential pregnancy

- **Menstruation** – both progesterone and estrogen are low as the womb lining is shed

That's the super-basic science of it all, but if you know *anything* about my work, you'll be aware that I care *much* more about the psycho-spiritual experience of the menstrual cycle – the energetic, emotional, spiritual, and psychological rise and fall that occurs as we move through each phase.

In each menstrual cycle phase, you experience life *through* the lens of that phase – in each one you feel, act, and show up to life in a different way. Interestingly, and NOT by coincidence, the phases of the menstrual cycle hold the same energetic frequencies as the phases of womanhood, the seasons, AND the moon, which makes the act of tracking and mapping them all a delicious act of Self Source-ery, a deepening of our roots, and a weaving of our own mycelium network into nature and the cosmos, *as* nature and the cosmos.

Getting geeky

Earlier, I alluded to how, at the age of 26, after years of misdiagnosis and bleeding more days than I wasn't each month, and wishing daily for a different body, I was diagnosed with endometriosis and PCOS. I was told by a doctor that I had zero chance of having kids so they might as well 'whip it out' (he was referring to my ovaries and womb).

Unfortunately, that doctor's response was/is NOT uncommon. Every week I hear from clients with menstrual and sexual health issues who have been told: 'There's nothing we can do – you're going to have to live/put up with the pain/heavy bleeding.' So many are prescribed the Pill as a way to 'manage' their symptoms, instead of having a health professional work with them, in the way I do, to get to the root cause.

I decided against the 'whip it out' solution, although I won't lie, I *was* tempted. Ultimately, I had a deeper knowing that there *had* to be more to it. That there *had* to be more choices and ways to heal and thrive, and not simply 'survive,' than taking synthetic hormones and painkillers, or having my reproductive organs removed.

So, I gave myself six months and I started to chart my cycle (something which, until that point, I thought only people who wanted to get pregnant did). I got geeky, charting everything from my temperature to the consistency of my cervical fluid; I also charted my moods, hot spots, and power points, when I wanted sex (and when I definitely didn't), when I was creative, when I could take action, and when I was more tired. In the process, I came into a relationship with both my inner and outer landscapes, my terrain, my magic, and my power.

The 'bloody' brilliant benefits

When you become familiar with your lived experience through the lens of your menstrual cycle, the following starts to happen:

- You begin to pick up on your body's cues (even the super-subtle ones).

- You recognize that the pain and discomfort you may experience is in fact a message that something deeper is going on for you and is wanting to be addressed.

- You become more responsive to your physical, emotional, and spiritual needs.

- You find that your *Red Journal* – this is the journal I created to track and map the cycle; you don't NEED this, you can make your own, but if you want something already created with love, by me, specifically for this process, I highly recommend it – and all the cycle intel you gather in it becomes your very own self-help book and life coach; there's more on journaling coming up later in the chapter.

- You begin to recognize that you can trust yourself to make smarter decisions and better choices and live your life in ways that feel creative, juicy, supportive, and nourishing to your lived experience.

Cycles within cycles

As I've said, ALL of these SHE cycles can be woven together – the seasons can be mapped onto the phases of the moon, the menstrual cycle, and the phases of womanhood. Cycles in cycles, on cycles, within cycles. THIS is the rhythmic intelligence of *all* things.

Through the first half of the cyclical experience – the phases of **Minx/pre-ovulation/waxing moon/spring** and **Creatrix/ovulation/ full moon/summer** – our energy is masculine. We're outward-focused and, like the moon as she moves from waxing to full, we're taking in a really deep inhalation as we grow and expand to meet the world.

Then, when we move into the second half of the cyclical experience – the phases of **Charmed** and **Dangerous/pre-menstruation/waning moon/autumn (fall)** and **Wise Crone/menstruation/dark moon/ winter** – our energy moves into the feminine. We start to turn inward, away from the world, and like the moon as she moves from waning to dark, we experience the deep release and let go of the exhalation as we retreat from the world and return home. To ourselves, to the Earth, to the void, to Ma of the Dark Matter.

So, the inhalation is masculine, filling us up with go-for-it, can-do energy, while the exhalation is feminine – a deep release, a slow-down and surrender inward. This beautiful masculine and feminine dance is happening in each breath, in our life cycle, in the phases of the moon, in the seasons, in the menstrual cycle.

Which is why, when you track and map *your* SHE-scape, you'll realize, quite quickly, that you have an opportunity to really KNOW yourself through an ever-changing spiritual, emotional, hormonal, creative energy that becomes a supportive map of YOUR landscape and your cyclical Self Source-ery.

Take it s l o o o w l y, and place your attention where you're most fascinated, knowing that at any one time there are many cycles within cycles occurring that you can access and look to for support in understanding, knowing, and loving on yourself better.

It's revolutionary. Literally.

Cyclical energetics

In the table opposite and the detailed intel that follows it, I've shared how each SHE cycle can and might look, feel, and be experienced, archetypally and energetically. I've also included the cyclical Self Source-ery that's available in each one, so as *you* map *your* cycles, you'll have an idea of how each one *might* show up for you and what potential magic is accessible to remember there.

Don't forget, though, that everyone's experience is different. I'll tell you what *I've* discovered – everything from tarot and elemental correspondences to what *I* need in order to feel fully sourced and vital, whether I'm tracking the moon, my menstrual phases, my womanhood phase, or the seasons – and then, as you explore the cycles yourself (through whichever cyclical lens you choose), you can start to make notes and tune in to what you need to align and self-source in sync with *your* natural rhythms and cyclical nature.

NOTE: If you've read any of my previous books, what follows may feel like known and familiar territory. Good. See if you can allow yourself to soften and go deeper. To let MORE of your own knowing and wisdom become present.

SEASON	🌱 SPRING	☀ SUMMER	🍁 AUTUMN/FALL	❄ WINTER
Lifecycle/ phase of womanhood	Minx – curious and sensual	Creatrix – fertile and fecund	Charmed *and* Dangerous – untamed and without a filter	Wise Crone – all-knowing, and cares very little for societal expectations
Magic Mistress-ry phase	Meet your magic	Begin mistress-ry of your magic	Mistress-ry of your magic in action	You are the mistress of magic
Moon phases	Waxing	Full	Waning	Dark
Menstrual cycle phase	Pre-ovulation	Ovulation	Pre-menstruation	Menstruation
The cyclical Self Source-ery available	Growth – plant new seeds and tend them Curiosity – open to new experiences and willing to try new things	Creation and manifestation – turning dreams and ideas into reality	Revealing – seeing everything exactly as it is Shedding – letting go	Death and rebirth – surrender and new beginnings Dream time – visioning
Feelings	Optimistic Daring Anything's possible	Self-assured Positive Confident	Sharp tongue No bullshit Discerning	Soft Dreamy Contemplative

NOTE: These are my interpretations of the archetypes and the energies held within them. I've re-imagined them from more patriarchal models; so, for example, as you read about the Minx, you might think, *Wait, that wasn't how it was for me at menarche*, or as you check out Charmed *and* Dangerous you may feel so bloody exhausted from having to navigate a world that is NOT set up in your favor that the idea of mistress-ing your magic is one you can't even entertain.

That's OK, my interpretations are simply a seed of wild hope, planted with love amongst these pages to support the remembrance. You can make up new words for each phase of your life and your cycles. In fact, I highly recommend it. In the same way that so many parts of a woman's body landscape are named for the men thought to have 'discovered' them – do NOT get me started on THAT – we get to reclaim and rename. You, on your terms, remember?

⏺ *Minx/pre-ovulation/waxing moon/spring phase*

Element: Air

Energy: Masculine and outward

Superpower: Being creative and taking risks

Mantra: 'I get shit done'

Tarot card: The Fool

Song: 'Like a Virgin' – Madonna

Minx

The Minx is fresh, young, and full of hope, possibility, and potential. She's frisky AND she's risk-taking. She's dynamic, active, and radiant. Like Kamala Khan in *Ms. Marvel*, or Dorothy in the movie *The Wizard of Oz* – who finds herself stepping onto a yellow brick road in this incredible new world of technicolor – she's naïve, wide-eyed, and a little trepidatious, but the possibilities of what's to come are palpable as she sets off on her new adventure.

However if, like me, during your Minx years you were (rudely) NOT crowned prom queen, or you didn't have the swishy just-stepped-out-of-the-salon hair, or maybe your first sexual experience was less than ideal, or your first bleed held a lot of shame (or it was a total non-event that's meant you have no relationship with your bleed AT ALL), there may be some subconscious angst or pain that makes this phase less than OK for you.

JOURNAL PROMPT

You may currently be in the Minx phase of womanhood, OR it may be a distant memory. You may be the mumma of a Minx and are having to relive and negotiate the terrain through her eyes. Or perhaps you're feeling the pressure of societal expectations to live up to the Minx ideal of beauty.

What does the word Minx bring up for you? What comes to mind when you think about puberty, your first bleed, your first kiss, your first sexual experience, your appearance at that time?

Magic Mistress-ry

It's here where we first meet our magic, where we encounter our body and its potentiality for growth and creation, and where we experience our influence and impact on others. We shape and form experiences from what we learn, and for many of us that's based on society, school, media, and familial teaching. But what if it was based on remembrance and mistress-ry of our magic? It would be here, as the Minx, that you'd meet it, play with it, inevitably mess up, but through trial and error recognize, for the first time, the source power that you wield and yield.

Waxing moon and pre-ovulation intel

Because your energy levels are rising, this is the phase where you can get work done, start new projects, go on dates, plant new seeds, try something new, and basically take advantage of the renewed energy that's flowing through you. It's a powerful time to take a leap of faith, take risks, and make big changes in your life. In this phase, you CAN produce to societal standards (because the systems and structures have been set up that way), but the question is, do you *want* to? And if you *do*, what do you want to create?

Spring wisdom

The Sabbat (an ancient pagan festival based on the Celtic Wheel of the Year) of Imbolc marks the onset of spring: after the death and darkness of the winter, we're all given the chance for a brand-new beginning, to start afresh, to plant new seeds and watch them grow.

Cyclical Self Source-ery

Here's what I've discovered is available and accessible in this phase:

- **Play** – experiment and let joy and lightness be present in the possibility.

- **Passion and enthusiasm and curiosity**. What for? ALL. THE. THINGS.

- **Sensuality** – taste new things, try new things, take a class that fires you up.

- **Growth** – socialize and surround yourself with people who encourage you to grow.

- **The opportunity to mess up** – in fact, I highly encourage it. Try things out, mess up, dare to be imperfect. Let the phase when you meet and keep re-meeting your magic be the place for trial and error, NOT perfectionism.

- **Take risks and take action** – in this phase it's way easier to do the 'risky' thing – like pitch a book, date someone new, make art for the first time. Say yes when you'd usually say no. (And if you don't like it, WHATEVER it is, exercise your absolute right to change your mind at ANY moment.)

- Turn off your phone and go on adventures. Have ALL the adventures.

◯ *Creatrix/ovulation/full moon/summer phase*

Element: Fire

Energy: Masculine and outward

Superpower: Confidence and self-assurance

Mantra: 'I can do ANYTHING (but that doesn't mean I have to do everything).'

Tarot card: The Empress

Song: 'Girl On Fire' – Alicia Keyes

Creatrix

Like the full moon when she's ripe and has reached her full potential, when you're in your Creatrix phase, you become your most full, fecund, and fertile and are able to manifest the seeds that were planted by the Minx.

It's a time when you become pregnant with life, but you don't have to become a baby mumma to be a Creatrix. This is when you're at your most creative and productive. You're also at your most sociable and your most expressive. And *these* combined? Well, they're the key ingredients for manifesting the very best kind of life magic.

As so often happens with powerful women in movies and myth, in the Marvel media franchise, the character Wanda Maximoff, the Scarlet Witch, is portrayed as 'mad.' Yet she has the power to create from will, and she does. Like her, *you* have the capacity to become the mistress of both your magic and your destiny.

JOURNAL PROMPT

For you, what does the word Creatrix bring up? Would you use something different?

Are you a mumma? If not, how does the phase usually associated with THE mother feel to you as Creatrix?

If you are a mumma, how does it feel? What does that word evoke in your being? Does it feel similar to or separate from the Creatrix?

What is currently wanting to be created through you and by you? How could you use the energy of this phase to harness your power and manifest your magic?

Magic Mistress-ry

It's here that you begin the mistress-ry of your magic. Where you recognize in the light of the full moon the capacity of your source power and how it can be used. So, it's here that you begin to gain mistress-ry of it. It's here that you begin to hone and harness the gifts and talents of your magic and source-ery.

Full moon and ovulation intel

During this phase it's WAY easier to network, to show up, to express yourself and your ideas and, more importantly, make them happen. You become magnetic, self-assured, and it's much easier to be confident (as in *really* confident, not bravado) and outward-facing (in the sense that you're happy to talk and be seen) than in any other phase. You're capable of forging deep connections and making lasting impressions now. If you want to ask for a raise, give a presentation, or have a deep talk with your partner, *this* is the time to do it. You are fire.

Summer wisdom

The ancient pagan Sabbat of Litha marks midsummer, the height of summer. It's the time of year when the crops are growing, and the earth has warmed up. Days are long and we can be in nature, socializing and spending time with others.

Cyclical Self Source-ery

- **Creation** – making, manifesting, and birthing (and rebirthing). Also, if you DO bleed, make yourself some meals while your energy is at its peak and freeze them ready for menstruation. The Wise Crone in you WILL thank you.

- **Expression** – through your voice, through your art, through the clothes you wear, the way you spend your time, the words you speak, who you spend time with. It's the mark you choose to make and the decisions that you take in alignment with your heart and belly, fully expressed in the world.

- **Illumination and visibility** – your gifts and talents are heightened, and as the Creatrix, you have the capacity to be seen, to share them articulately and with confidence.

- **Being effective** – look, you *can* get shit done in this phase. (It doesn't mean you have to.) You may have a tendency to push too hard – the productivity spell we've ALL been put under is strong – which will inevitably lead to burn-out. Your energy levels are high, so use them wisely.

● *Charmed and Dangerous/pre-menstruation/ waning moon/autumn (fall) phase*

Element: Water

Energy: Feminine and inward

Superpower: The ability to cut through bullshit

Tarot card: Lust

Mantra: 'Do not underestimate me. I *know* myself'

Song: Respect – Aretha Franklin

Charmed *and* Dangerous

The masculine, logical, straight-line thinking and practical traits that served us as the Minx and Creatrix now become a very limited toolkit as we enter the feminine-led phases. There's a distinct energetic shift from 'doing' to 'being.' Unfortunately, we've been told that we can, and *should*, simply keep on pushing through and functioning and producing at the same level of high energy.

Only, just as it is when we experience a menstrual cycle, just as it is when the energy of the moon begins to wane, that's simply NOT possible. At least, not without some serious side effects, which can range from irritability, frustration, confusion, and sadness through to depression, anxiety, addiction and burn-out.

As I mentioned earlier, this phase in our lived experience is often overlooked, which I find particularly interesting because it represents all that's wild, charmed, AND dangerous – she's the Lust card in the tarot, the version of womanhood that modern society ignores in favor of a younger and more vital version. We can witness this play out in Angelina Jolie's portrayal of the villainess fairy Maleficent in the movie of the same name.

Yet, it's here that we have a deep, intuitive understanding of the universe, where we care much less about the mundanity of life and instead turn our attention to the mystical. We cultivate the wisdom and insight from our lived experience and remembered knowing and we use this to teach, share, and nourish rather than to try to control and manipulate.

NOTE: This is indicative of the virtually never-talked-about phase of perimenopause – see why I called this phase Charmed *and* Dangerous? *Perimenopause* is such a disempowering word; in fact, it lacks ANY kind of power – which is the transitional period between our bleeding years and menopause. Naturopath Dr. Vera Martins, in her blog for Mpowder.store, describes perimenopause as 'a time of heightened hormonal instability. It's like your hormones are on a rollercoaster – think of it as a reverse puberty.'

Because it's rarely openly spoken about, perimenopause has many feeling that they're going 'crazy,' which is also how many of us feel each month as we experience our pre-menstruation phase. We've been tamed, shushed, and censored and that's never more present than in this part of our life AND this phase of our menstrual cycle. Because it's here that our wildness – our truth, our voice, our bodies, our very essence, in all its messy imperfectness – demands to be untamed and uncensored. Now, if that *actually* happened, we'd become less compliant; we'd see through the societal lies and deception and well... that would make us 'dangerous.'

The Charmed *and* Dangerous phase *should* be where we feel most at home, yet we've been taught and told to go against our cyclical nature, so we inevitably suffer. We become so disconnected from our knowing that we no longer recognize how to return to it. It's time to remember and reclaim ALL that's potent and powerful about this phase.

EXTRA NOTE: I'm often asked if I'll write a book about perimenopause and menopause, and the answer is yes. As I navigate it, finding tools and rituals and rites that support me through my own particular rite of passage, I'll share those with you. Promise.

JOURNAL PROMPT

What does what I've shared about Charmed *and* Dangerous evoke in you?

What emotions are present when you feel into this phase? Are you rageful? Are you scared of what it would mean to be both charmed AND dangerous? Or do you recognize yourself here?

Do you suppress what is charmed and dangerous in you? Does she feel so uncontrollable that you have to keep her on a leash? Or do you feel trapped and want more than anything to feel her expressed through you?

When I first explored my Charmed *and* Dangerous self, I was scared of her. I thought she was 'too much.' My magic, me, connected to source, seeing it ALL – well, that felt WAY too much. But that's what we've been programmed to believe. So, slowly, with each cycle, I took the opportunity to meet myself in this phase. I explored my rage, my uncensored nature, and turned bitchy-ness to bitchcraft. And I've harnessed it – not tamed it – so that I can really put it to use. So that *I* can really be of use.

Magic Mistress-ry

In this phase all that was seemingly mundane becomes the terrain of the mystic. You've honed your mistress-ry – you KNOW your magic because you KNOW yourself and you're able to apply it, practice discernment about when and how to use it, and know when to turn it up and when to turn it down.

This is something I witnessed in my mumma. I KNEW she was magic because my nanna was magic, but they were both, my mumma especially, really scared that people would know they had it. When I was writing *Witch*, I didn't really get it – as the last of my matriarchal lineage I wanted that fear of persecution to end with me.

But as we navigate these current times, I understand more than ever HOW important it is for me to KNOW my magic, to KNOW how to harness my source power, to fortify and self-source AND to be able to recognize and discern when to turn it all the way down too. Our mistress-ry is in really bloody KNOWING that we are both Charmed *and* Dangerous and to act accordingly.

Pre-menstruation and waning moon intel

This is a move into the terrain of the feminine: an invitation to stop going so fast, to produce less, and instead turn inward and be open to receive. If you allow this, and don't resist it, it creates SO MUCH clarity. You may feel the need to clean, decorate, or tidy the house, organize your office and filing system, and edit people and negative situations out of your life. Be warned, anything you swept under the carpet/chose to ignore in the first half of the cyclical experience will often reappear in this phase. It's a time for analysis and discernment.

Autumn (fall) wisdom

The ancient pagan Sabbat of Samhain marks autumn (fall). The time of year when the trees start to shed their leaves, when you feel the need to be indoors more, preparing for the winter. It's an invitation to look inward, to care less about what's going on in the outside world and instead, turn your attention to your own inner landscape.

Cyclical Self Source-ery

- **Inner sight** – when we slow down and turn inward, we can connect to our pythoness power, source power, so much more in this phase than any other. (It doesn't mean we can't connect in other phases, it's just much more heightened here.)

- **Harvest** – celebrate and have gratitude for all that you have.

- **Edit and discern** – both tolerance and levels of patience can be low in this phase, but your ability to cut through bullshit will be high.

- **Truth-seeking** (of both your own truth and that of others). Your bullshit detector is turned ALL the way up, and you will demand authenticity and all that's real (again, from yourself and from others).

- **Break down old beliefs and ways of thinking.** Yep, anything that doesn't feel like it's supportive and nourishing is dismantled, and it's where real feminine repair can occur.

● Wise Crone/menstruation/dark moon/ autumn (fall) phase

Element: Earth

Energy: Feminine and inward

Superpower: Heightened senses and an awareness of *everything*

Mantra: 'Let it flow'

Tarot card: World

Song: 'Time to Flow' – D-Nice feat. Treach

Look up the word 'crone' in the dictionary and you'll see the definition 'ugly old woman.' A hag. She's the one who was most feared in the 'woman/witch hunts.' Why? Because she KNEW the most.

She's old and she's wise. She represents the woman who's in menopause. (Again, I hate this word – can we create a new vocab for our experience, PLEASE?) We no longer have to experience each phase of the menstrual cycle because when we become the Wise Crone, we have, and hold, ALL the phases *within* us. We have an all-seeing perspective of the life-living experience. We are wisdom personified. We know stuff. We are between worlds – the veil is super-thin here, which is why our magic is so strong. The ancient-future ancestors are close and it's easier to converse with them here than in any other phase.

The Wise Crone, and this is one of the MANY reasons why I love this phase, is immune to bullshit and *should* now be able to live a life free of these constraints; although in Western society so many women enter menopause without any preparation, awareness, or knowledge of the power they hold there and can feel 'washed up' and as if they're no longer needed or required. (Because, conveniently, that's what's perpetuated through so much of the media we consume.)

Look for representations of this woman in your life. It won't be easy, as the media and society are even less fond of the Wise Crone than they are of the Charmed and Dangerous woman, but they are out there and when you meet them, you'll see they are bloody glorious. I particularly love Professor McGonagall in the 'Harry Potter' movies and Princess Leia in the 'Star Wars' sequel movies.

Connecting with the Wise Crone is connecting with the part of you that's infinitely wise, all-knowing, understanding, and compassionate, yet also direct, to-the-point, and with absolutely categorically NO fucks to give.

JOURNAL PROMPT

How do you feel about getting/being older? Is there fear? Concern? Excitement?

What was/is your relationship with the Wise Crones in your family? Did you know them, did you spend time with them? What stories of theirs are you currently carrying? Do you need to continue carrying them? Are they a legacy or a burden? Do they need to be celebrated or released?

Magic Mistress-ry

In this phase you fully embody your magic – you are the Mistress of your magic. There's nothing left to remember, you are IT. Why, in the fairy tales, is the old crone portrayed as an 'evil' witch? Because it's when we are at our MOST powerful.

Menstruation and dark moon intel

This is the phase in which to connect with your inner wisdom. In fact, if you let it, this is an opportunity for deep reflection each month, a chance to release what's no longer necessary and relevant in your life and to really get a feel for what's necessary and relevant moving forward. That way, you can dream, vision, and remember, so that you can plant the seeds of your visions, dreams, and remembrance as you move back into the pre-ovulation/waxing moon phase. Smart, huh?

Winter wisdom

The ancient pagan Sabbat of Yule marks midwinter, the dark before the light, that darkest moment – and we've all experienced those, right? The dark night of the soul, which brings you to your knees and makes you think you'll *never* experience light again. Yet we celebrate this cyclical winter solstice, the day each year with the fewest hours of light, because we know, with total certainty, that the light IS returning.

This is what happens with our menstrual cycle in the days before we bleed. It calls us toward the dark, asks us to be willing to let go of what no longer serves us; and when we do bleed, there's both release and relief as we cycle toward the light of ovulation – midsummer – once again.

Cyclical Self Source-ery

- **Dream and vision** – I mentioned earlier the 'dreaming womb' in the Hypogeum in Malta, a temple created specifically for women to dream creation into being, because they took 'dreaming' VERY seriously, and so do I. Let your dreams, specifically at the dark of the moon or during menstruation if you bleed, be a sacred vision time. Allow for visions and downloads to take shape in the space of NO thing, where EVERY thing is possible.

- **Tend** – brew your favorite tea and eat chocolate – I love ceremonial cacao AND I love milk-y sweet rose.

- **Cook** – if you bleed, you'll be thanking your Creatrix right now for batch-cooking you nourishing meals for when you're in this place and space between worlds.

The how-to-track-and-map bit

Look, while I'm pretty sure that you don't NEED me to tell you *how* to journal, I *have* created *The Red Journal* for those who are interested in mapping and tracking the moon and/or the menstrual cycle (you don't have to menstruate to benefit from it). However, if you're someone who likes to freestyle, here are some of the things that you *could* chart daily in your journal:

- The date

- Astrological sign

- Phase the moon is in

- Astrological sign the moon is in

- Season

- If you bleed, which day of your cycle you're on

- The Feels – you can chart your emotions: how you're feeling, physically, mentally, and spiritually. Your energy levels: how well you slept and for how long. Your mood; your dreams; your relationship to others; your sex drive.

- Self Source-ery – you can chart your wants, needs, and desires. Where's your head at? What movement did you do today? What movement would feel good? Where have you experienced pleasure? What would you need today for pleasure to occur? What did you do to nourish yourself? What would feel good that you haven't done already?

- Heart Riffs – simply riff with your heart about what was positive and what was challenging that day. What came up for you? Did you react or respond?

You can make this a super-detailed daily exploration or create a simple legend of symbols that are unique to you and *your* process. Then, at the end of each month (or moon cycle, menstrual cycle, or season… you get the idea), you can turn super sleuth, go back over your journal entries, and pick up cues and clues about what's actually going on for you IN your body from cycle to cycle.

NOTE: Let YOUR unique-to-you rhythmic intelligence make itself known to YOU. Maybe you're called to pay more attention to your sleep and dream patterns – for example, our circadian rhythms are in sync with the sun, which also has an impact on our insulin/blood-sugar balance, hormones, gut health, sleep, and mood.

Or if, like me, you menstruate and are astrology obsessed, track and map which astrological signs you bleed in and which astrological sign the moon is in when you bleed (because every month, she moves through each astrological sign approximately every 2.5 days).

This intel has created a deepening in my own knowing, and it means I care less about the 28ish-day cycle and much more about the astrology of that particular cycle. If you're called, I really recommend it (and if you want to explore it further, I offer a self-study 'bloody astrology' online program – www.thesassyshe.com/bloodyastrology).

Life-living as a cyclical exploration

I'm a BIG fan of journaling, but honestly, my hope is that you make exploring YOUR SHE-scape a playful experience, and that in the process, you discover lots of insight and intel about yourself that helps, supports, and guides you to:

- Remember your magic.

- Know, trust, and listen to YOUR natural rhythms through your own lived experience.

- Cultivate self-trust – your cyclical nature helps you to trust your all-seeing, all-feeling, true nature. To trust your belly-deep pythoness to move you toward or away from situations/people/places without logic, and yet knowing that the reasons will unfold and reveal themselves.

- Practice – through the cycles, seasons, and rhythms – the act and art of receiving care and nourishment. Honoring where you're at in any given moment and meeting, tending to, and nourishing yourself there by creating more body-honoring rituals and fewer goal-orientated routines.

- Take action (or not) based on your own self-knowledge – based on YOU and YOUR needs – so that you can live in right relationship with it ALL.

What if you don't bleed?

Or perhaps you're experiencing perimenopause or period irregularities? Wherever you are on the delicious spectrum of being human, wherever you're at in your lived experience cycle, the ever-constant that so many temple priestesses before us turned to, worked with, and ritualized, was the moon.

So, if this cyclical Self Source-ery is new to you, or you don't experience a menstrual cycle, my advice? Attune with the moon. Each moon cycle, we get the opportunity to wax and wane with her rhythmic flow and plug in to and amplify the teachings and learnings of each phase. It's seriously beautiful and powerful stuff and it's the ONLY thing I can trust, which is why I share this non-linear, can't-be-taught offering to support YOUR cyclical exploration.

Contradictions and inconsistencies

The energetics of the cycles at play at any one time can, and will, sometimes feel in opposition to each other. This can create discomfort and have you questioning, 'Er... which cycle should I actually be following?'

For example, there was a six-year period when I experienced my menstruation at full moon, so in my body I felt the need to slow down, rest, shed, and regenerate, while at the same time, the moon was at her fullest, encouraging me to be out and seen in the world. It felt like a 'push me, pull you' sensation where my inner landscape was at odds with the outer landscape.

So, I leaned into it and got curious about what I could potentially discover there. The result – apart from it initially being really bloody annoying – was that I built a personal resilience: an inner ability to adapt and shapeshift between inner and outer landscapes that I wouldn't have recognized had I not been tracking and mapping my SHE-scape.

NOTE: Look, this *is* the realm of feminine magic and mistress-ry, so it's not always pretty and it's never straightforward. (That's the idea.) But as we all look to navigate the uncertainty and chaos of These Times, our SHE-scape creates that much needed grace-space to practice fortification, understanding, repair, and compassion.

For everything there's a season (and a reason)

In the same way that the seasons change and the moon waxes and wanes, so too do our moods, our creativity, our energy levels, our appetite, our sexual needs – *all* the things. Remember and recognize that time is NOT linear, and that creatively and emotionally, physically and spiritually, we can be starting a cycle, in a cycle, and ending a cycle at any one time AND at the same time.

For example, when you find out you're pregnant, you begin a new cycle with growing and birthing your baby as your focus. Or when you reach menopause, you start a new cycle exploring your place of power. Or after becoming single for the first time in what feels like forever, you move house and change jobs, and so you start a new cycle of navigating life differently. Or a trillion different versions of what happens when one cycle of being ends and a new one begins and how, at any one time, these beginnings and endings are all overlapping.

It's why there is NO formula.

It's NOT a formula

When we develop a felt sense of our cycles and rhythms, we disrupt the systems and structures that have us believing we're machines that need to produce and always be on, available, and accessible to the point of exhaustion. We're being called, in the reclamation of our source power, to remember our magic. To self-source through our own lived rhythm and cyclical nature.

But it's NOT a formula; I repeat, it's NOT a formula. (Although it's as close to one as I'll ever get.) It's a practice/process/art form that replicates nature in that it KNOWS there are no deadlines, to-do lists, and goals to achieve; instead, there are periods of growth, transition, action, gestation, blooming, shedding, death, stillness, and rebirth.

When we KNOW where we are and what's available to us in each space, place, time, and phase, we know that for every season, there's a reason. We know what we can work with and how to leverage it energetically; we know what may make our life a li'l trickier and mean that we have to grow strong roots, stand taller, be more adaptable; and we also know what will give us the support we need to show up, exactly as we are. Unapologetically.

Cycles in cycles,
on cycles,
within cycles.

This is the rhythmic
intelligence of
ALL things.

The Venus Vortex

I don't know if I've mentioned this, *ahem*, but I'm a massive enthusiast of exploring the cosmic and astrological cycles and alignments and their impact on the body. I also mentioned earlier that my matrilineal lineage, Gypsy/Traveller, was/is 'sky readers,' which basically means we're not interested in the angles and degrees of astrology as such, but 'feel' the planets and constellations. We understand their correspondences with the seasons, with herbs, body parts, and nature, and we literally read the sky's story *through* the body.

So, for me, embodying the planets, the stars, and the wisdom is WAY more powerful than learning the very complex language of astrology (which I have done, am doing, and will continue to do – but mostly, I like my way better. Ha!)

The Empress

Since my mumma died, my Ma quest of Self Source-ery has had me coming deeper into communion with the Empress archetype. Now, I share this because the Empress card in the tarot is ruled by the planet Venus, and Venus as Empress holds fierce feminine medicine. Her links to Mary Magdalene, the wild rose, and the Egyptian temples of Isis, and Hathor before her, have taken me on some of *the* wildest adventures.

And as I've tracked Venus's cycles, in alignment with my own Venus cycle (in alignment with the cycles of ALL the things), it's become super clear that so much of our work as women in this lifetime is to re-vision and retell Her story through OUR bodies and OUR experiences.

The Empress is a mumma, but not necessarily a mumma of children.

She's a leader, but not in an old paradigm-y patriarchal way.

She's powerful, potent, and beauty-full, but not in a conventional sense.

I 'met' the Empress intimately when I was asked to lead a retreat. As is the case with all my retreats, I was gifted a title for it, but not the bloody content – no matter how nicely I asked and no matter how hard I tried to bloody plan. The title? The Empress Codes. Now, the tarot is heavily loaded with archetypal symbology and information and intelligence, so I turned to the Empress card. But even the cards in my favorite tarot decks didn't hold the potency and power of the Empress I was evoking *through* my body.

This woman was POW-ER-FULL.

Bold.

Strong.

Potent.

Whole.

Not in an armored, keeping-it-together-so-no-one-can-see-I'm-actually-falling-apart way, but in the way that only a woman who KNOWS herself and really feels herself IN that knowing can. She was Cleopatra, Lizzo, AND the Queen of Sheba. So, I drew her. (Making art, direct from the heart, is how I started to make sense of it all. I was very much a do-it-in-secret art splasher until my mumma died, then on her death, I claimed space as a bold mark-maker who channels SHE through my coloring pens. You can find the finished Empress card in the *SHE Sirens Oracle* deck. AND yes, you better believe that as I'm writing *this* book, there's artwork for a *Self Source-ery* deck moving through too – I cannot wait to share it with you.) And through *my* version of the Empress, the work became clear.

The Empress is our way back to our power.

The empress often represents pregnancy and birth. Now, this doesn't have to mean a baby, although it certainly *can* mean that. More often, though, like the archetypal Creatrix, it refers to our potential to create and give birth to ANYTHING.

At that solstice, on that retreat, with the glorious women who had heard their own siren call and were gathered there with me, I began to birth more of who I was becoming.

The Empress.

My own mumma.

A woman who is fecund and fertile ground.

A woman who is IN her body and trusts herself as her own safe space.

Only, I got scared. Because to BE the Empress is to birth an entirely new possibility, and to do that, you REALLY have to die to all that you were previously. To all the ideas of who you think you should be. To what others expect of you.

All the old stories, all the old beliefs, my relationship with my body, with my mumma, my relationship with being a mumma, the grief, the death – all the death – the feeling of abandonment, of being unlovable, and who those stories and beliefs have made me, became suddenly MORE important than who I was to become.

But this particular cycle was already in motion, and years later, I'm still becoming. I'm perpetually becoming.

Becoming my own safe space.

Becoming my own mumma.

Becoming my own power source.

Becoming my own force. (For goodness, sensual pleasure, THE GOOD STUFF.)

Which is *how* Venus and her cycles became my THING.

The Venus cycle

Y'see, you may know Venus as the goddess of beauty and love in both Greek and Roman mythology; you may know her as a planet in the night sky; you may know her as an ancient statuette or relief of the feminine form, such as the Venus of Willendorf or the Venus of Laussel. But there's *SO* much more to her than that. SO. MUCH. MORE.

You need only look at the delicious dance that Venus, the Earth, and the sun participate in to create the sacred geometry of both a five-pointed pentagram and a wild rose to *know* that Venus holds some powerful and potent Divine Feminine wisdom.

Her astrological symbol, often called a 'mirror,' is a key to unlocking her whispers and her mysteries within you. If you're called, draw it, and pin it to your wall or in the front of your journal; or ink it onto your skin with a Sharpie; or place it on your altar – and connect with it daily.

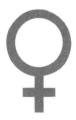

The Venus symbol

Cosmic hook-ups

Each Venus cycle – a cycle is roughly 19 months long – I work with women in the SHE Power Collective (an online community that you're so welcome to join: www.thesassyshe.com/shepowercollective) to connect with Venus through her monthly encounter with the moon. In each lunar cycle, Venus and the moon meet in what some call a 'portal,' some call a 'kiss,' and others call a 'gate'; personally, I call it a cosmic hook-up.

While the new and full moons connect us to the lunar feminine and anchor us into our emotions, our unconscious, and our conditioning, the cosmic hook-ups between the moon and Venus as she circles the sun align us with the evolutionary frequencies of what astrologer Sasha Rose calls the 'solar feminine,' and they offer us *another* cyclical map with which to orient our month.

A SHE quest

If, like me, you're called to go deeper into this Venusian portal, know that Venus offers us a cyclical rhythm to reveal the hidden mysteries of the initiatory ascent and descent journey of Venus/Inanna.

Venus, like the ancient Sumerian goddess Inanna, who is also known by many other names and for many things, including love AND war, takes us on a shamanic journey, a SHE quest. As Venus makes her descent as the morning star, for seven months, each cosmic hook-up – the time each month when Venus and the moon are conjunct – represents a descent IN to the body, from the crown chakra to the root chakra. If you're willing.

Each cosmic hook-up is an arrival at a chakra descending deeper IN to your body. An opportunity to strip yourself of anything and everything that isn't your truest expression with regard to that chakra representation. So that when you arrive at the 'metamorphic underworld' (when Venus moves toward a conjunction with the sun, which means she's no longer visible in the sky, for approximately 40 days; hmmm, where have we heard THAT before?) at the root of *your* being, it's here that you 'die' to What's Been Before and all that you thought you were. So you can re-member and re-birth wiser and rooted IN your power.

Because, just as Venus does when she drops below the horizon as the morning star to be reborn as the evening star; just as the moon does when she wanes into darkness only to appear a few days later as a waxing crescent; just as you, if you bleed, move from pre-menstruation into the darkness of menstruation so you can be rebirthed ready for a new cycle of unfolding, Venus has built-in periods of 'death,' a time out for processing, and this is where you can access what REALLY matters.

Descent into the dark

In the most famous telling of the story of Inanna, she descends into the underworld, where she meets her sister, Ereshkigal, who is queen of the underworld. And for us, taking the journey alongside Inanna, this is where we enter the void.

It's here in the depths of the cosmic cauldron that we're able to meet the dark feminine. To spend those 40-odd days while Venus is no longer visible in the sky entering into the deep, dark woods, stripped of all we thought we were, looking to reclaim ourselves. The places and spaces where parts of us have been exiled, hidden, suppressed, and repressed. Our bite. Our power. Our courage. Our knowing. A remembrance that here, in the dark, is where you/we came from.

I ESPECIALLY love the cyclical map of Venus because so many of us avoid the darkness, preferring to stay in the light, make a peace sign and shout 'positive vibes only.' That's great until an event or situation comes along that takes you out at the knees and you're *not* prepared – physically, mentally, emotionally, spiritually – for how to navigate the dark places.

This cyclical map is of a journey we can *choose* to take. It's a conscious shedding, like the serpent, of that which no longer serves us. A release of all the things we 'think' we need but which actually restrict us – all the places we fight and resist.

We retrace Inanna's steps, and we enter into the darkness of the underworld and surrender. While in the story Ereshkigal hangs her sister on a meat hook – good news, you DON'T have to do that – we can take this time, in the void of the cosmic womb, to really know ourselves in the dark.

Who are YOU as the dark feminine?

In this space, I remember all the parts of me that I've disowned in order to be likeable, nice, and 'good.' My rage, my magic, my mysticism, my passion, my most true and real expression have *all* been exiled here, in the darkness, at one stage or another, in order to be 'accepted' and 'likeable':

Don't talk about THAT – they'll think you're crazy.

Don't act THAT way – they'll think you're too much/too loud.

Don't have an opinion – they'll judge you.

And when I DID come belly-to-earth with the dark feminine in me – and I'm not talking shadow, I'm talking simply about the opposite of light: dark, that which is necessary, in fact, totally required, for us to be whole – she demanded to be reclaimed and revered.

So that I honor my rage as sacred and holy.

So that I no longer fear death.

So I know that in the dark, the chaotic, and the unknown I shed, I grow. I menstruate. I thrive.

And then, just as day follows night, we return. Back up, through the body, through the seven chakras from root to crown, claiming, honoring, and revering at each monthly cosmic hook-up between the moon and Venus, what was revealed to us in the dark.

And, just as it was for Inanna in the story, you'll find that you don't return from the underworld full of love, light, and all things sugary sweet. No, it's the same when they talk about the morning star, Venus, being the 'light bringer' – the light that's brought, when alchemized in the underworld, is stripped-back and without-filter TRUTH. (Imagine if we were all able to create and share from THAT place!)

My journey with Venus and Inanna began in the darkness of my mumma dying. As with every heroine's journey, it's rare that the descent from power and safety is ever voluntary; in fact, a rapid descent often occurs on THIS particular path, when someone the journey-taker loves is taken from them. The Venus cycle, however, offers us an opportunity to actively *choose* to enter in. So that when we inevitably *do* find ourselves in the darkness, because we will, we KNOW it.

We know who we are there.

We no longer fear it.

We know what's possible there AND we also know that we can and that we do return.

NOTE: If you're interested in going deep with the Inanna mythos, I recommend you start by reading *Inanna* by Diane Wolkstein – SO GOOD. My favorite line? 'She applauds her vulva for being so wondrous.' LOVE IT.

Now, before we move on, I want to briefly introduce you to another female powerhouse:

Meet Enheduanna

Enheduanna was an Akkadian high priestess who, it's said (and quite honestly, I'm ALL about it) is the earliest author known by name. And what did she write? Incantations, prayers, stories, and song. Sigh. The most famous was 'Nin Me Sara,' a sacred song to the goddess Inanna. She wrote it while in exile, and it led to wars being won and eventually to her liberation. Now THAT is word power, witches.

Enheduanna wrote lots of hymns to Inanna, the Divine Feminine, celebrating her relationship with her. I'm obsessed, and I introduce you to her because through her relationship with Inanna she strengthened her relationship with herself, who she was, and what she stood for and believed in.

So, my invitation to you is to, like Enheduanna before you, create a devotional to Venus/Inanna. It's through *my* devotion to Her, the descent and the ascent, the shedding and the becoming, that I'm able to recognize myself as sacred and worthy of self-devotion. I wish that more than anything for you, too.

Invitation
A Venusian devotional

I invite you, in true temple priestess style, to light a candle, spray your favorite perfume, or diffuse oils or burn incense, play a sensual song of your choice, and gently move your body – sway, swirl your hips – and as you do so, track your sensations, track your pleasure.

✯ *Seek the pleasure. Follow the pleasure as you move your body.*

✯ *When the song finishes, imagine and vision that you're now in a sacred temple – feel, sense, and experience yourself there.*

✯ *Place your hand on your heart space and imagine that what lies beneath the palm of your hand is a beautiful emerald. Bring your attention down into this place and space.*

✯ *Take your hand away from your heart, pick up a pen, look out and through your emerald heart and write to her, to Inanna, to Venus, to you at your most sacred, through the lens of the heart. Write a love song, an incantation, a poem to SHE. To the most divine and sacred part of YOU.*

The best day to do this practice is a Friday because that's Venus day. You can also dedicate Friday as a celebration and devotion to YOU. Buy yourself flowers, wear your most sacred scent, diffuse oils, wear your favorite ensemble – lavish yourself with the most delicious love. Worship yourself as you'd worship the Divine.

...

Devotion over
discipline.
(Every single time.)

Know Your Flow

In each place and space, within each cyclical experience and rhythm of life, you have access to insight, codes, and wisdom that *can* and *will* help you to make 'sense' of, get clear about, and enhance your fully lived experience.

It's self-revealing. Self-replenishing. Self-revitalizing. **It's Self Source-ery.**

The practice of tracking and mapping cycles – aligning and syncing their rhythms with our lives and nurturing an ever-unfolding, intimate relationship with the source power that's revealed there (which also takes into account the complexities and nuances of our daily lives) – gets under the skin, under conscious awareness, and creates a deepening.

A soul-deep remembering that our ancient cyclical and rhythmic intelligence is source magic for These Times.

Not consistent, but cyclical

Yep, the cyclical experience offers up rhythms that support, nurture, nourish, and provide an amazing opportunity for you to align and live in sync with them. To be in flow. YOUR flow. Knowing that EVERYTHING has a season (and a reason), and that these rhythms are in relationship with and inform one another, means you're able to cultivate a fierce and loving, ever-evolving relationship with yourself, your magic, and your power.

You begin to pick up on your body's cues (even the more subtle ones); you can recognize pain and discomfort as a messenger that something deeper is going on; and you become more responsive to your physical, emotional, and spiritual needs.

When you know why you do the things you do, why you act a certain way at certain times of the month or year, that there's a season for your reason, you begin to breathe a little easier.

You're less hard on yourself, you heal – physically, emotionally, psychologically – you reclaim power, sovereignty, and agency over your body and your lived experience and, despite what you may have previously been told, you realize that you're *not* crazy. You realize that you're *not* consistent, either – you're cyclical, with a unique-to-you-rhythm, vibration, frequency, and song. And that's a GOOD thing.

SHE RIFF – LIVE YOUR RHYTHM

With your feet firmly rooted into Mumma Earth, take a deep breath, release any contraction and tightness you may currently be feeling in your body and be open to the possibility of expansion.

Be open to the possibility that there's more available to you than you know. (Except you DO know.)

Be open to the possibility that things are happening EXACTLY as they should.

Be open to the possibility that life is working in your favor.

Be open to the possibility that you get to
cocreate your reality with the cosmos.

It might not feel like that, and that's OK
– all I'm asking is that you allow yourself
to be open to the possibility.

Can you do that? Can you be here, in the present moment?

Can you also see that you're a part of something
WAAAY bigger? As above, so below.

When you remember and recognize that you have your feet
firmly on Mumma Earth in the present AND you have access
to all that's been and all that's to come, you'll KNOW,
your deep inner gnostic knowing will know, that rushing,
doing, reacting is NOT what's required right now.

The world needs your creative pulse and
response to be in collaboration with the
cycles and the rhythms of the cosmos.

The Earth and stars meeting in every one of your cells.

You have the power to choose (always)

Let go of the ideas and plans and structures that your human self
feels the need to hold on to tightly in order to justify its existence on
Earth. When you do, you'll breathe a little deeper, you'll release the
grip on that particular reality, and you'll remember that you have the
power to choose.

**Choose to let the cyclical container initiate, innovate, grow, and
potentize your Self Source-ery.**

Because then, there's a new possibility – one of innovation, where
YOU initiate and cocreate reality. Not to the exclusion of your human
experience. You're *not* bypassing, you're *not* making a peace sign
and taking a selfie, although you totally can – you, on your terms,

remember? You're in recognition of the humanness AND you're in recognition of your cyclical rhythms and magic. You create and respond, and it's medicine for you and it's medicine for the collective.

High fives and deep bows to THAT.

When the drummers were women

'The sky and its stars make music to you
The sun and the moon praise you
The gods exalt you
The goddesses sing to you.'

These words are inscribed on a wall in the Temple of Hathor in Dendera, Egypt, and alongside them is an image of one of my favorite deities, the Egyptian Mumma goddess Hathor – SHE who represents women, fertility, pleasure, dance, and the arts – playing a frame drum.

As the late Layne Redmond – drummer, author of *When the Drummers Were Women* and one of my incredible teachers – so beautifully articulated, 'In the ancient world, from Turkey into the Mediterranean, in Egypt and the Middle East, the drummers were women.' These women drummers were priestesses of both Death and Creation – they were in service to Ma.

In many traditions and cultures, you'll find that the women would wear their hair wild and loose, and drum. They'd drum in celebration, they'd drum in ceremony and ritual, AND they'd drum (and lament and wail) to awaken the souls of the dead for their journey to the underworld. (The drumming would also awaken the souls of those still living to help integrate their grief as a community.)

Many of the temple priestesses' drums had a dot painted in their center, a *bindu*: the symbol of the compacted, unmanifested energy of the universe before the first sound. Others were painted blood red. Now, the first sound that we hear in the womb is our mumma's blood pulsating through her arteries, so to paint a drum red, or to put a *bindu* at its center, represented everything – the potentiality – before it comes into existence.

The sacred act of a woman/priestess banging/stroking/playing the drum is a symbol of woman as Creatrix of the universe.

One stroke of the drum, and EVERYTHING comes into existence.

INVITATION
YOUR RHYTHM, YOUR RULES

Read the words in bold below:

Can you remember the time when the drummers were women? A time when the frame drum was a ritual instrument? When it was used to celebrate life, to support the dying and death process, and to encourage rebirth, regeneration, and creation in all its forms?

A time when the beat of the drum represented the rhythmic intelligence held within a woman's body and celebrated her as a Creatrix, a powerhouse, a Source-ress? (It's no bloody surprise that women's drumming as part of spiritual and religious life was banned, is it?!)

Now, if it feels safe for you to do so, close your eyes, breathe into your belly, and on the exhale, let your attention drop past your heart, past your belly, and into your pelvic bowl. With each inhale and exhale, let your body soften and listen for the beat of the drum. It's ancient. You know it. Feel, sense, and experience yourself in this vision.

Where are you? How does it feel?

I've immersed myself in this energetic transmission for years now. One where the ancestral mother lines, from all the different cultures and traditions, meet in the mistress-ry of the mystery and drum: to move the grief, to honor the dead, to celebrate life, and to do the work of this lifetime – repairing and regenerating the feminine, the Ma frequency in ALL humanity.

So, the invitation is to come and meet me in the dreamtime of this. My hope is that we dream it into a real-time experience where we are ALL drumming and singing, together, with the ancestors past and future here in present time and across timelines and paradigms, cocreating What Comes Next.

• • •

Follow the beat of *your* drum

Currently, there are entire universes lying unmanifested and dormant in your being. So, what's moving through YOU that needs to be created? What's begging to be realized? When you remember that you're a Source-ress who can bring anything into being when you tune in to the beat of YOUR drum – YOUR big, beat-y heart, YOUR unique-to-you frequency, YOUR rhythm and flow – you no longer need to follow anyone.

It's easier to be in action because YOU set the pace.

Your rhythm, your rules.

You, without all the false programming.

You, connected to your passion, creativity, courage, confidence, and capacity to love.

You, with your intuition, senses, and inner sight activated and turned all the way to full.

You, connected to the source of life itself.

Yep, you're a vibe, and your frequency is your siren song, and your siren song is Divine source power ACTUALIZED.

She bangs

I often have wild dreams and visions of my lifetimes spent in Hathor's Temple, drumming, dancing, and shaking a sistrum, so it's no surprise that I'm a drummer in *this* lifetime too. When you're of Gypsy/Traveller descent, there's very little escape from the beat of a drum or the rattle of a tambourine. My uncles used to play frame drums in pubs on a Sunday night, and I would drink lemonade, eat a bag of crisps, and swirl, twirl, and dance until I was dizzy.

When I was 11, I played side drum in a marching band (I KNOW!). I now play the tambourine, sistrum, and frame drums in ritual and ceremony, in sacred spaces, to clear space, to manifest dreams into being, to go on shamanic journeys (and I'm not going to lie, it's also REALLLY good when you're angry and need to let out a whole lot of frustration, to simply bang the shit out of a drum. RARRR!)

It's how I stay connected in my body to my own rhythmic intelligence and how I connect with the rhythmic nature of Mumma Nature, the moon, and the cosmos.

You don't need a drum to remember that your rhythmic intelligence is a creative force, a power that can initiate, innovate, heal, and transform, but drums ARE an incredible medicine tool. (You can come make one with me and the Viking – we run sacred frame-drum-making workshops: www.thesassyshe.com/shebangs – VERY powerful!)

> Our rhythms and our connection
> to the rhythms of nature and the
> cosmos are a FIERCE source power
> in navigating the current terrain.

I've found that the more I tune in to my cycles and the wisdom they hold through that distinct-to-me beat, the less need I have to 'follow,' compete, or compare myself to others. Yes, it's hard when there's so much bloody noise, but it IS possible, and the more you make space to listen, the less fear-fucked you become. Actual fact.

FYI: I DO NOT have this totally figured out. It takes time. I've had to/still am ALWAYS learning to really lean into faith and self-trust. Trusting that doing things to the beat of my own drum, my siren call, and *not* what everyone else is doing, WILL pay off.

Ultimately, when I keep plugging into Mumma Nature, and when I reconnect to the cyclical and rhythmic intelligence of all things, I build trust with the beat of MY drum. My unique-to-me truth frequency. AND I wish that for you too.

Your unique-to-you drumbeat

Now, can you trust that each of us has our own unique drumbeat? Our own rhythm which, like the moon, the seasons, and the tides, ebbs and flows and guides us in the right direction?

There's a chance, since you're here in this cauldron of Self Source-ery, that it may feel as if your beat and rhythms go against the flow of other people's – and oh, how we want to be like the others, right? (Keep recognizing where all the 'good girl' tendencies STILL show up and remind them that there's NO place for them here.)

When you listen and trust your own drumbeat, the rhythm that's unique to you, you'll begin to realize that everything's unfolding exactly as it should. That's not to say you should sit back and let life happen to you, but when you trust your own rhythm, life becomes a collaboration – you know *when* to create, rest, nourish, be in action, and you trust that it may not be in sync with others. And you trust THAT too.

What does *your* drumbeat sound like? What is its rhythm? Is it slow and sultry with a hot and heavy pounding? Or is it graceful and light, and make you want to pirouette in a tutu? Maybe it's erratic and loud, demanding that you shake your ass?

Recognize that this can be different in each phase of the moon, and in each and every moment, because different seasons, life phases, and stages may dictate a different beat. So, take time each morning to breathe deeply, move your body, and check in with your own frequency and beat.

Ask yourself:

'What's my rhythm today and how can I honor it?'

'How can I dance with it? How can I lead from that place?'

Remember (and *keep* remembering)

Whichever cycle, phase, and rhythm of life you're currently experiencing, I'm so glad you're here. Even if, right now, it feels incredibly painful. Even if, right now, the idea of disconnecting, numbing, going along with what you've been told and sold for a perceived easier life feels WAY more appealing.

FYI: If this *is* how you're feeling, I'm sending you ALL THE LOVE – I STILL find that I disconnect VERY easily (*The Real Housewives*, anyone?!) There's NO right way to do this, and the many of us who DO feel it all are also feeling the bigger collective pain, fear, and uncertainty. And that? Well, THAT can be all-consuming.

How do *I* build and maintain that reconnection and trust with my instinctual knowing?

I remember.

I remember that it's a mother-loving process. Literally.

I remember ancestral Ma. The wisdom held in our bones and belly and cells.

I remember my visions and dreams of an ancient-future.

I remember a place of KNOWING that cannot always be articulated and made meaning of.

I remember (and honor) my body and her rhythms.

I remember (and honor) the Earth and her rhythms.

I remember (and honor) the cosmos and her rhythms.

So, if you *do* disconnect, if you *do* forget to remember, let yourself get underneath your own skin and trust that hope still holds strong. When I/you/we resonate at our unique-to-us frequency, we come into the sweetest alignment with ALL THAT IS. A new field of possibility arises, and it calls us, like the Source-resses before and yet to come, to dance.

Please, let's dance.

Dance, move, alchemize, and re-sensitize

I've never quite shed my previous life as a temple priestess (who would want to?), which is why I LOVE to participate in the art of burlesque and belly dance. But my BIGGEST love? It's to put on a curated playlist and let my body f e e e l what it's feeling and move, un-choreographed. Moving my body to release, alchemize, re-sensitize.

In the same way that they were drummers, women have ALWAYS used dance as medicine and magic. Not to please others (although I've no doubt that it did and does that) but to charm their own serpentine flow with hip swirls and belly ripples. To activate their own source power as healing, magnetic, and regenerative magic. (Might they have used this movement power to 'charm' others and to bend and shape certain outcomes? I imagine so, and high fives and titty shimmies to THAT.)

Dance, singing, and music have been used since the beginning of time to generate healing. The Hathor temples in Egypt, Ggantija in Gozo, and remember the tarantella? It's *all* my muse. As a trained somatic practitioner and Movement in Practice facilitator, my IN.YOUR.BODY.MENT® classes and workshops are curated spaces – not to 'get fit,' although you 'might,' but ultimately ceremonial places where you can come, check in with your SHE-scape, and move, dance, sweat, pray, co-regulate your nervous system and cocreate the support you need, in that moment, through breath, sound, and movement.

Dr. Peter Lovatt, author of *The Dance Cure*, is one of my favorite humans and I'm honored that I get to call him my teacher. He says: 'Humans are born to dance. In today's sedentary world, we would all benefit from doing more of it. Science shows that just 10 minutes of dancing provides a thorough workout for the body and brain, raising the heartbeat to cause a release of feel-good endorphins, connecting us to our emotions, and reducing our stress levels. Dancing quite simply makes us feel more alive.'

We're not sideline observers. Each and every one of us has a place and space, a voice in the divine orchestra, a heart in the great rhythmic dance, and we need to reclaim our space on the cosmic dance floor.

How? We reconnect with all the rhythms in all the ways. We move. To the beat of our own drum. Not the one that we've been told and sold, but the unique-to-us beat of our own heart and belly and pelvic bowl.

To the siren song held in the oceanic yearning and learnings of our being in connection with the Earth and the cosmos – this is Ma consciousness, this is source-ery. Creatrix power. And it's here that you get to deprogram, unravel, and detangle. To return to the truth of the pythoness and dance.

Dance the dance of YOUR rhythmic intelligence.

Remembering, reconnecting, and reclaiming in fierce reverence.

You are the magic and medicine of THAT vibration. THAT frequency.

And you/I/we will be unapologetic about it.

As we dance. Dance. Dance.

Because in the dance, I become more me, you become more you, and we become WE.

Aligned.

Magnetic.

Whole.

Don't dance as if NO one's looking, dance as if EVERYONE is watching.

⟡ YOU, self-sourced ⟡

YOU remember. Your magic *through* your body. You can see in the dark, smell the fox scent of your knowing, feel the rhythm of your drumbeat, and sing your siren song.

YOU know that through your body, your rhythms, your voice, your song, and your frequency you *can* find ease and freedom and liberation. (On your terms. In your own time.)

YOU remember your cyclical nature and allow yourself the space (of grace) to flow. (On your terms. In your own time.)

YOU have faith and trust that when your body is met and seen in the fullness of *your* expression, in ALL of your seasons, that the places and spaces that have got really used to protecting and defending you can soften, and you can let your body become magnetic, fertile, fecund, sacred ground where magic- and medicine-making is omnipresent. (On your terms. In your own time.)

YOU rest AND you bloom. You nourish AND you flourish. (On your terms. In your own time.)

YOU recognize that it's time to bring it all together and devote yourself to *your* mother-loving true nature. (On your terms, and in your own time.) AND you also recognize that by doing THIS, you undo centuries-old societal spells that have tried to keep you from this very remembering.

YOU know that ALL life is a process of becoming and that you are ALWAYS becoming that which you already are. Because... paradoxes, remember?!

Live your rhythm.

What Now?

Self Source-ery is *your* magic and medicine.

It's ever-unfolding cyclical support.

It's not performative, it's devotional.

It's presence without pretense or persona.

It's you, IN your body, in the mistress-ry of the mystery.

Self Source-ery – just saying the words out loud evokes the deep knowing of the pythoness, doesn't it? – is body magic, which is why everything I've shared within these pages carries a vibration, a transmission, a frequency, alchemical in nature, that WILL unlock memories, (g)knowing, maps, songs, and codes to support you in navigating *your* own journey and experience of life.

Not the conventional Joseph Campbell-created 'hero's journey' that we're familiar with and which plays out in *all* the movies. Not the journey we've been sold as self-development, where you become better, more perfect, and quite possibly more 'righteous.' No, this is a *different* journey, one that's shaped and formed in a way that's rarely, if ever, been templated to us before, because a woman in remembrance of the cycles and rhythms of her mother-loving true nature is deemed 'dangerous' to the systems that benefit from keeping us tame, keeping us quiet, keeping us compliant.

A labyrinth walk

This is a labyrinth walk. An invitation to come in and come down, where the 'wicked' witches and 'dangerous' women are actually Source-resses. Women who KNOW. Who are potent, magnetic and perpetually birthing more of who they are here to become.

They know that their song, their siren call, is in their blood and bones. It's in the waterways of their being, it's in each and every cell, waiting, wanting to be sung and expressed through them.

This is a journey where:

You're allowed (and also you don't need ANYONE'S permission) to be magnetic and fecund ground for magic and miracles AND witness the war, greed, and destruction in the world.

You're actively encouraged to support, nourish, and give to others AND be supported, nurtured, and nourished yourself. YOU REALLY ARE.

You choose to mother yourself, to grow yourself up, and to take radical responsibility for your action and your choices.

You can feel and sense the full spectrum of emotions and sensations without wanting to disconnect instantly. (You still might, but your capacity is super s t r e e e t c h y.)

You can hold a variety of perspectives (along with their complexities and nuances) without having to prove that you're right and others are wrong.

You know there's no goal. There's nothing to fix. There's nothing to get 'better' at. The ONLY outcome is simply to keep revealing *more* of who you are.

You're present to, and really good and OK with, EXACTLY what 'is.' To source vitality and aliveness, at source, so that, slowly and tentatively and with a shit ton of love and compassion, you can expand your capacity to hold more.

It's a journey that goes deep into the belly of your being, gets dirt under your fingernails, can really bloody burn (in order for you to learn and discern), and often takes the longest way home. (Because integration and recalibration CANNOT be rushed.)

FYI: There's no destination. This journey is a lifelong labyrinth walk – in and down, up and out – perpetually birthing *more* of who you already are.

THIS is the revolution.

NOTE: A revolution happens when cycles are fully experienced, completed, learned from, metabolized, and alchemized.

Self Source-ery completes and supports the revolution of cycles, so that we don't get stuck in fear and/or trauma. It's a process. Ongoing. Lifelong. No beginning, no end. Continually aligning, refining, and redefining. With curiosity and endless fascination. Allow it to bring direction to all that you do and all that you are in the world.

Self Source-ery is not another 'thing' on your to-do list. It's not a reductive and prescriptive bullet-point plan on care and life-living. It's a prod and a wink, direct from source, to evoke and provoke a FULLY LIVED EXPERIENCE that expands and deepens your self-knowledge – your senses, your intuition, your instincts, and your magic.

Cyclical awareness = self-knowledge
Self-knowledge = self-power
Self-power = full IN.YOUR.BODY presence
Full IN.YOUR.BODY presence = YOU, SELF-SOURCED

A Source-ress – SHE whose magic, power, and wisdom are felt, restored, regenerated, and reclaimed In. Her. Body.

SHE who is fecund, nourished, satiated, and sourced, *at* source, *by* source, is fertile ground for *any* possibility of becoming. SHE can navigate, innovate, and cocreate a life, a fully lived experience, a world that is... well, really bloody glorious, and more importantly, really bloody necessary.

AND SO IT MOTHER-LOVING IS.

Closing Ceremony –
Own Your Throne

Source-ress, birth a new possibility.

One where you are NOT a result of the story you've been told about yourself by others, by your family, by society.

One where YOU are powerful.

YOU are potent.

YOU are fecund.

YOU are fertile.

YOU manifest. (Everything from new life to creative projects, to entire fucking universes.)

One where you're no longer waiting to be saved or rescued.

One where you DO give a fuck, but you're VERY discerning about where, and to whom, you give those fucks.

One where you're not seeking approval or validation.

One where you're not waiting for someone to buy you a ring or find your clitoris. (Mainly because you can buy your own, and you can DEFINITELY bring yourself to orgasm.)

Because from your root to your crown, you are sovereign and it's time to own your throne.

∼ THE CEREMONY ∼

WHAT YOU'LL NEED

A bowl; rose petals or salt (optional); rose essential oil; spring water (or tap water that you've blessed with your own choice of whispered words); your journal and a pen; a mirror.

WHAT TO DO

If it feels good, cast a circle – using either a pointed finger, rose petals, or salt – and step into it. Call on your spirit team to be present (ancestors, spirits, animal totems, or guides), ask for protection, and declare your space open.

✶ Take a breath, deep into your heart and pelvic bowl, and release it noisily. Do this five times. Feel yourself dropping an energetic anchor deep down to Mumma Earth.

Breathe in, and push energy down into Mumma Earth, through your medicine bowl, through your roots, and into HER roots. Breathe out and pull energy up into your roots, from HER roots, and into your cauldron, your sacral space. If it helps, place a hand there.

✶ Do this practice for a few minutes in silence. When it's complete, open your journal and ask yourself:

'Who am I? Who is this woman who's being called to own her throne?'

Let your heart and belly riff on the response. Feel, DON'T think. When complete, fill the bowl with the water and into it, make a declaration about yourself, the woman who's being called to own her throne.

Something like, 'I... (your name) **am a Source-ress of Power and Pleasure and Potency and I...** (choose words that are specific to your own passion, pleasure, and purpose), **and I own my throne.'**

Repeat your declaration three times. The water holds your words; now drink it down and allow the declaration-infused water to work through you.

✱ When you're ready, fill the bowl with water again and add a few drops of the rose oil.

Stand, and dip your thumb in the rose water; repeat your declaration and place your thumb at your forehead.

Pause.

Dip your thumb in the rose water, repeat your declaration, and place your thumb at your mouth.

Pause.

Dip your thumb in the rose water, repeat your declaration, and place your thumb at your throat.

Pause.

Dip your thumb in the rose water, repeat your declaration, and place your thumb at your solar plexus.

Pause.

Dip your thumb in the rose water, repeat your declaration, and place your thumb at your pelvic bowl.

Pause.

When complete, take the mirror in your hand, stare at your glorious reflection, at the woman you are, at the woman who's claiming her throne, and make your declaration to your reflection one last time.

✫ Close your circle, thank your team for their protection and support, and declare your space closed.

• • •

Remember, reconnect with, reclaim, and revere your power.

Your power to self-source.

Your power to perpetually birth and become *more* of who you are.

Do it for you, do it for those who have walked the path before you, with you, and for those who are yet to come.

Own your throne
and crown yourself
a sovereign
Source-ress.

Acknowledgments

High fives, chest bumps, and deep bows of love, chocolate, and appreciation to:

SHE. Always. Thanks for being the ULTIMATE Source-ress. For helping me to return home – over and over again – to my body, to my truth, to my magic, through you, as you, and to perpetually keep birthing my own becoming. I love you.

The SHE Power Collective: you glorious gathering of women are the reason this book and the medicine held within it exists. Your support and your big, beauty-full, beat-y hearts, our Moonday card-pulls together, our reads of the SHE-scape and rituals and ceremonies helped me to re-member. MY voice. MY art. MY magic. You have been, and continue to be, THE most delicious space to be a woman in process. Loves, we are the Source-resses. This time is OURS.

The Hay House team: you're ALL so bloody brilliant.

Michelle, thanks for trusting my instincts and magic and for being a real and true force of nature.

Debra, your patience and 'rigor' created the perfect container to hold the chaos of my creative flow. BIG LOVE. Lisette – thanks for your expertise, sensitivity, and big, beauty-full heart.

My love fam: the Viking – my bearded forever love. Whatta life, eh? I'm so glad we're doing it together, hot husband. I BLOODY LOVE YOU. Leanne and Sarah – the Best by name AND by nature – I do NOT know what I did to deserve you both in my world, but I'm really bloody happy, grateful, blessed for it. Nicholas, Aimee, Katie, David, Mary, Jenny, and Karen: thanks for being my people. My loves, my friends, my emotional support humans, food feeders, WhatsApp message-ers, space providers, meme sharers. ALL THE THINGS. I LOVE YOU.

To Carrie-Anne, Eleanor, Evanna, LeAnn, Leanne and Maude – thanks for your realness, your big hearts, your work in the world, and your support. Honored that I get to know and love you.

Oh, and to the team at Rowdy and Fancy's for making THE most delicious and magic Sweet Rose chocolate bar – not an ad: I paid a LOT of money for ALL THE CHOCOLATE I ate as I wrote, and I do not regret it ONE BIT. (In fact, you may be the reason this book actually got finished. So, THANK YOU.)

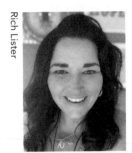

Rich Lister

About the Author

Lisa Lister is a best-selling author, artist, oracle, well-woman therapist, somatic movement teacher and practitioner and a Movement in Practice facilitator. She offers practical, psychological, and spiritual tools, guidance, space, and support to women who are exploring, navigating, and healing their relationship with their body, their cycles, their sexuality, and their power.

www.thesassyshe.com

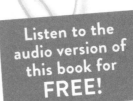
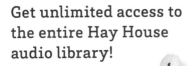

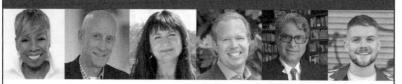

CONNECT WITH
HAY HOUSE
ONLINE

 hayhouse.co.uk   **f** @hayhouse

 @hayhouseuk   @hayhouseuk

 @hayhouseuk   @hayhouseuk

Find out all about our latest books & card decks • Be the first to know about exclusive discounts • Interact with our authors in live broadcasts • Celebrate the cycle of the seasons with us • Watch free videos from your favourite authors • Connect with like-minded souls

'*The gateways to wisdom and knowledge are always open.*'

Louise Hay